LOOK
YOUNG
LIVE
LONGER

Also by Glenn Harrold

De-stress Your Life
Sleep Well Every Night
Lose Weight Now!
The Answer

LOOK
YOUNG
LIVE
LONGER

**A new approach to
reducing the signs of ageing**

Glenn Harrold

First published in Great Britain in 2009 by Orion Books
This edition first published in 2019 by Orion Spring
an imprint of The Orion Publishing Group Ltd
Carmelite House, 50 Victoria Embankment
London EC4Y 0DZ

An Hachette UK Company

1 3 5 7 9 10 8 6 4 2

Every effort has been made to ensure that the information in the book
is accurate. The information in this book may not be applicable in each
individual case so it is advised that professional medical advice is obtained
for specific health matters and before changing any medication or dosage.
Neither the publisher nor author accepts any legal responsibility for any
personal injury or other damage or loss arising from the use of the
information in this book. In addition, if you are concerned about
your diet or exercise regime and wish to change them, you
should consult a health practitioner first.

A CIP catalogue record for this book is
available from the British Library.

ISBN 978 1 4091 8558 1

Designed in Swift Light by Geoff Green Book Design, Cambridge
Printed and bound in Great Britain by Clays Ltd, Elcograf S.p.A.

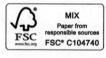

www.orionbooks.co.uk

Contents

Step 2 – Exercise and fitness

Step 3 – Positive mental attitude

Step 4 – Healthy sleeping patterns

Step 5 – Financial security and career contentment

Step 6 – Relationships

Step 7 – Spiritual well-being

Introduction

Welcome

'A man is not old as long as he is seeking something.'

Jean Rostand

The obsession with health and beauty these days seems to be worldwide. Television programmes, magazines and movies bombard us with images of 'beautiful people' – those blessed with inherent good looks, fabulous skin and flawless bodies. The newspapers are full of stories – good and bad – of men and women who have opted for plastic surgery, breast enhancements, Botox injections, hair transplants, or undergone other radical physical transformations in their quest for eternal youth. Popular programmes like *Ten Years Younger*, *Extreme Makeover*, *You Are What You Eat* and *Fit Club* fill television schedules, as well as those featuring celebrities offering branded items of clothing that lift, flatten and slim. The message often seems to be that – for a fee – you can halt the ageing process, knock years off your perceived age and join the ranks of the beautiful virtually overnight.

The idea of a quick fix is especially appealing in these days of fast everything – from food to sound bites – and high-pressure modern living with its constant messages to improve, acquire and achieve. If you are one of those who feel left behind by all this striving, or whose self-esteem has dipped because of a breakdown in a relationship, worries about the future, poor health or the sense that you have lost your youth, then the lure of the surgeon's knife, a jab of a needle or the popping of a pill can become disproportionately alluring.

Even more relevant to how you look or feel, though, is how you are in terms of your physical and mental health. Obesity is at an all-time high, levels of diabetes and heart disease are soaring, and studies have repeatedly linked cancer and other serious illnesses to lifestyle, stress and diet. We are bombarded with conflicting information about what we should or shouldn't eat, how much we should exercise, and where or how we should live. I am not a nutritionist and I do not earn my living as a fitness instructor or a medical expert or even as a statistician. I am, however, a firm believer that we are all in control of our own destiny as far as our well-being is concerned. Through my own experience, I know that it is possible to enjoy great health, rarely fall ill, and slow the ageing process completely naturally. There is no magic potion for this, but if you are willing to make some adjustments to your lifestyle then you can achieve this *easily* and for free.

I will show you how. Follow my seven-step programme in this book, be true to the changes you have decided to make in your life, and I guarantee you levels of vitality and energy that you thought possible only for someone in the flush of youth.

Even though I am in my mid-fifties now, I am far fitter than I was thirty years ago. Through my own hard lessons, I have learnt how to completely alter my own body's metabolism and become incredibly fit and healthy. I will share those experiences with you and show you how you, too, can stall the ageing process, unleash your own potential, and achieve optimum health.

I will teach you not only how to make these adjustments, but how to *enjoy* them by helping you create a positive mindset. Before long, being fit, healthy and positive will feel entirely natural to you, and you'll wonder why you didn't do something like this sooner. Enjoying the process is the key to long-term success and my programme is designed to help you achieve precisely that. So throw away the magazines, turn off the television, and focus on yourself instead of everyone around you. If you genuinely want to live a longer and healthier life, then now is the time to step up to the mark and make that commitment to yourself.

Every day that passes without taking these positive steps is a day wasted. You deserve nothing less than optimum health and longevity for however many years you have left on this earth. This is your divine right. Here is your chance to claim it.

My story

My start in life was anything but positive. I had a difficult and largely dysfunctional upbringing that left me with all kinds of problems. By the age of twelve, I was often sleeping rough on the streets – not the easiest of options, especially in the middle of winter in south London. At such a tender age, it was particularly tough, but the more it happened, the more I grew accustomed to it. Years later in a therapy session, my unconscious mind threw up a suppressed fear of the cold. At first I didn't understand where it could have come from, but after further analysis I was able to trace it straight back to those freezing nights.

My young life continued to be full of trauma. On my fifteenth birthday, I drank fifteen pints of beer in a single day – one for every year of my life – and collapsed in a stupor. A few months later, I was expelled from school for disruptive behaviour. I got involved in street fights; I lived on a Romany site for a while and had several run-ins with the law. At sixteen I was beaten so badly by a gang outside a bar that I was left unconscious and had to be hospitalized. The next two years passed in a blur of binge drinking, heavy smoking and delinquency, but then, unexpectedly, there came a glimmer of a future for me when I taught myself how to play the bass guitar and started a punk band called The Vagrants. Adapting to the changing culture of the early Eighties, we smoothed down our spiky hair, took off our rings and studs, and morphed into the more pop-based Sugar Ray Five, from which time we suddenly took off. Having won the Battle of the Bands, a national music competition with a prize of ten thousand pounds and a recording contract, we looked set for stardom.

Unfortunately, our overnight success evaporated as quickly as it had materialized, but not before we were introduced to the world of serious drinking and drug-taking. When I was seventeen, I woke up one morning barely able to move. My skin was bright yellow. A doctor diagnosed hepatitis and told me I would be dead with eighteen months unless I gave up drink. Fortunately, I saw sense, took his advice and for the next year survived on a diet a rabbit would be proud of. My healthier choices and abstention from alcohol allowed my young body to make a full recovery. It was an early lesson for me in how you can turn your life around by making a positive choice.

I didn't seem to take enough heed of it at the time, however, because in my late teens I acquired a new addiction – drugs. I experimented with all the usual mind-expanding suspects up until my early twenties. As you can imagine this unpromising start didn't do me much good either. Quite apart from the damage I must have been doing to my body, drugs messed with my mind and any career plans I might have had. True to all predictions, by the time I reached adulthood, I bombed. I was unable to hold down a job and everything I touched turned to stone. I was permanently broke, my relationships with women were brief, and I spiralled into an abyss of loneliness, depression and apathy. Married young, and with a new baby to provide for, I took a series of jobs driving delivery vans or mini-cabs. Needless to say, my marriage broke up after just a few years.

Writing songs and playing music had long been my only salvation, so for seven years I earned a living playing covers in pubs, clubs, bars and restaurants. I met a singer called Aly who became my second wife, and we formed a duo appropriately called Wishful Thinking. On the cabaret circuit year in year out, we often shared the bill with a stage hypnotist who invited people to come on stage so he could hypnotize them to do silly tricks. I had always been fascinated by the power of the mind and, watching his show one night, I had an epiphany. I decided that I wanted to learn everything I could about hypnosis, not to create a stage show but as a way of helping people in a career diametrically opposed to show business.

Having used up the last of my savings on the most comprehensive clinical hypnotherapy course in Britain, I spent the next two years intensely studying when not playing nightclubs and bars at evenings and weekends. At the end of the course I passed my exams with flying colours. It was the first time I'd passed anything since the eleven-plus. Despite the warnings from my tutors that only five per cent of graduates went on to make successful careers out of hypnotherapy, I borrowed a thousand pounds from a bank and set up a small private practice. Clients soon started trickling in, in greater numbers as word spread, and I began treating them for everything from anxiety to nightmares and phobias.

I gained immense satisfaction from being able to use my new skills. I helped so-called 'problem kids', those wanting to lose weight, people who were desperate to give up smoking, stop drinking, or quit indulging in obsessive–compulsive behaviour. Using hypnotherapy, I helped clients overcome sleep problems, their fears of flying or spiders, to relax and build their self-esteem. I learned that we each have so much talent, brilliance and determination inside us that all I had to do was open up people's minds to harness their own ability, creativity and imagination to develop a powerful and lasting self-motivation.

Drawing on my recording industry experience, I began to create hypnosis tapes for my clients to take home and reinforce the good work we had done. Combining my knowledge of music and hypnosis, I devised hypnotherapy sessions which included subtle background sounds recorded in certain keys and frequencies to enhance the effect. Initial feedback was amazing. People seemed to like my straightforward approach, which didn't rely on psychobabble or impenetrable phraseology. Whenever my tapes and CDs sold out, I duplicated some more and drove all over south London and Kent delivering them to book shops, chemists and health shops. Sales continued to snowball, so I set up my own publishing company to market and distribute them. My wife Aly became my business partner in the venture. Within three years we were so busy that I needed to take on full-time staff.

Studying my bank statements one day, my accountant queried a direct debit to my bank. Looking at the figure, I couldn't help but laugh. The thirty-six pounds per month was paying off my original thousand pound loan. I had completely forgotten about it, probably because that year alone my company turned over more than five hundred thousand pounds.

Twenty-five years on from the days when I was almost dependent on drink, cigarettes and drugs, I am completely free of the destructive urges that drove me to such excesses. I realize now that those bad habits were caused by a need to escape the memories of my childhood. I look back on that young delinquent and barely recognize myself. Two decades on, I am completely in tune with my life and my body and have found an equilibrium and level of fitness I could only dream about back then. Challenging myself daily has given me courage and confidence. I am now a non-smoking vegetarian who drinks only the occasional glass of wine. I have the same twenty-eight-inch waist I had in my teens and have made a conscious effort not to develop a spare tyre or 'man-boobs' like so many middle-aged friends and acquaintances. Having built up my immune system, I rarely get colds, flu, headaches or other common ailments. I swim regularly, play tennis three times a week, practise yoga and use self-hypnosis and meditation to achieve my personal goals.

I am a devoted father to Lee. My first wife Kim is still a close friend, and my publishing company employs ten fabulous staff. I have become Britain's best-selling self-help audio author with millions of sales of my hypnotherapy books, CDs, apps and MP3 downloads worldwide. My hypnosis audios are the UK's best selling self-help ranges of all time, with more than 10 million sold, and via iTunes, the App Store and other platforms my titles have also become one of the world's most downloaded self-help series.

There was a great deal of negativity in my early years, but through self-help therapy and determination I transformed that into positive energy to make a success of myself. Best of all, in turning my world around I have massively improved my own life expectancy and now enjoy the rude health, glowing skin and physical fitness of someone ten or twenty years younger. Much of my therapeutic approach to problem-solving has come from my own experiences, not from regurgitating text books or watching television programmes. Harsh lessons, such as those I learned struggling through my adolescence, gave me the kind of understanding of life, plus compassion and empathy for others, that can't be taught. When you have walked a tough path and overcome obstacles by yourself, you become a natural teacher and the best possible example. Having trodden that difficult path and chosen myself a better one, I feel more than well qualified to show others how to succeed.

Re-programming the mind

'Every man desires to live long, but no man would be old.'

Jonathan Swift

Have you ever committed to a new healthy lifestyle with enthusiasm and resolve, only to slip back into old, destructive patterns three months later? For many people, the answer is yes. One of the reasons for this is that even the best weight loss and health programmes only teach you to eat healthily and exercise on a *conscious* level. The only way to guarantee lasting commitment to any new pattern of behaviour is to re-programme your mind, and not just the part of the mind that deals with your conscious self.

Experts believe that the conscious part of our brain accounts for only around ten per cent of our mental capacity. It seems such a waste to cart a big, heavy brain around and then fail to make full use of it. You are going to achieve your lifestyle changes by learning to tap into the larger, creative and more resourceful part of your brain. The key to this is through the inner worlds of meditation, visualization and self-hypnosis. This is where your innate power and creativity lie. As you may already have realized, working on a health goal on a superficial, conscious level doesn't always create lasting change. To succeed in the long term you also need to work at a deeper, *unconscious* level.

Better still, by tapping into these unconscious levels, becoming fit and healthy doesn't have to be a struggle anymore. If you don't feel good as you achieve your goals, your willpower may falter, so enjoying the whole process is vital. When you re-programme your thought processes through hypnosis that is exactly what will happen. You will feel great about yourself *and* learn how to develop a powerful new self-esteem, giving you real motivation to be mindful of what you eat and drink, how much you exercise, sleep, or work on improving your relationships. Having a holistic approach to your health is the key to making lasting changes.

This programme can help anyone achieve permanent results. The only people who can't be helped are those who don't really want help, or who choose to wallow in their self-pity and neglect. If someone is unfit or unhappy with how they look or feel but can't be bothered to make the necessary changes to effect a transformation and give them a sense of self-worth, then there is nothing anyone can do to help them. Their attitude usually comes about as a result of negative conditioning in their past. The good news is that even if you have suffered such conditioning previously in your own life, you can still overcome it if you truly want to. It all depends how much you want it. Life-enhancing and life-affirming decisions have to come from within and you have to be truthful to yourself and your life goals. If you believe that you have that spark of desire – and the mere fact that you are reading this suggests that you have – then anything is possible.

Welcome to the rest of your life.

How hypnosis works

'The idea is to die young as late as possible.'

Ashley Montagu

Watching in the wings as the stage hypnotist persuaded a member of the audience that she was strongly attracted to a broom, while her boyfriend was convinced that he was Elvis Presley, left me in no doubt of the power of the mind. My interest, however, was always in how that power could be put to beneficial use rather than for comic or dramatic effect.

Probably the one question I am most commonly asked is, 'You're not going to turn me into a chicken, are you?' which has become a damaging legacy of stage hypnosis shows. People also tell me, 'I don't want to look into your eyes in case you make me do something strange,' or they use the expression 'putting me under', which implies that they won't be in control. This isn't true at all; they will merely be in an altered state of consciousness.

Don't let the thought of being under hypnosis scare you, as it is often misunderstood. Being hypnotized is neither frightening nor dangerous and it does not induce a false condition. Even if you think you've never been in a hypnotic trance state before, let me assure you that you have. Twice a day, every day, we are all naturally in a state akin to that induced by hypnosis – the 'hypnopompic' state when we are in the transition state of semi-consciousness between sleeping and waking, and the 'hypnagogic' state which comes on at the onset of sleep. In either case we are fully in control, just relaxed and more receptive to suggestion. Daydreaming is another naturally occurring trance state that is familiar to us all.

When you go to sleep at night and drift between

consciousness and unconsciousness, your brain-waves are actually slowing down. When you go into a hypnotic trance exactly the same thing happens, although you remain aware of your surroundings even as you drift into deeper states. It can sometimes feel as though very little is happening when you are hypnotized and that you can open your eyes at any time and be wide awake. This is true but you can still achieve lasting changes from being even in the lightest trance.

Now you can learn how to create those states at will to empower yourself and develop a healthy lifestyle. By reinforcing positive not negative aspects of your psyche, reiterating the good and conditioning your way of thinking, you will be able to tap into the unexplored regions of the brain where such suggestions remain long after hypnosis. Studies have shown that just by visualizing yourself doing a work-out, for example – running, swimming, or taking some form of exercise – your body can show signs of increased muscle toning and conditioning. Quite literally, you can think yourself fit. Imagine then, how much could be achieved if you could not only harness your own abilities to think yourself healthy and full of vitality, but also back up those commitments with a strategy to put it into effect. A man was recently cured of cancer by the injection of massive numbers of his own immune cells, grown in a laboratory and transferred back to his body to fight the disease. Doctors hope one day to find ways of promoting the growth of these cells *within* the body of the sufferer, using whatever means they can. As we continue to explore the depths of the mind and its hidden powers, hypnosis is one of the options being considered.

Imagine an iceberg with its tip above the water and the majority of its vast bulk lying beneath the surface. This analogy is often used to describe the conscious and unconscious mind. We spend most of our time in our conscious thoughts and only sporadically tap into our unconscious mind when we daydream or think creatively. The longest time we spend in our unconscious thoughts is when we are sleeping, when our conscious mind has switched off. Learning to connect with your deeper unconscious mind by focusing your thoughts can help you in so many different ways to achieve goals, find your creativity and overcome difficulties.

Throughout this book there are a number of self-hypnosis and visualization techniques, along with hypnotic affirmations, which will help you re-programme your mind. When you start to use them, don't worry if you feel you're not going into a deep enough trance at first. Affirmations and visualizations are a remarkably effective re-programming method and they will still make a big impact on your inner thought processes. Just by closing your eyes, breathing deeply and focusing on the affirmations as you say them, you will begin to make positive changes in the way you think and feel about your health and well-being.

How the book and audio download work

The different techniques in this book add up to a powerful holistic solution to help you become healthier in mind, body and spirit. Use those that are most relevant to your own situation. If your biggest problem is that you eat too much fatty food, for example, then pay more attention to the techniques that help you break free of bad eating habits. If you have problems sleeping, then focus more on the sleep section. If you have money worries or relationship difficulties that are dragging you down, be more mindful of the suggestions in those chapters, and so on.

The accompanying self-hypnosis audio download was created specifically to reinforce the messages within these pages (to receive the download go to www. glennharrold.com/orion/lookyoung). It is important you begin using the audio straight away. The hypnosis techniques and subtle sound effects have been carefully created for maximum impact, using certain keys and frequencies which help to guide you into a deep state of mental and physical relaxation. When you are in this receptive state, you will be given a number of post-hypnotic and direct suggestions to help you achieve goals that will help you to live longer and look younger.

I recommend you listen to the audio download through headphones while lying down, as this way you will absorb all the positive suggestions and affirmations on a deeper level. If you fall asleep while listening but still hear me count from one to ten at the end of the track, you have probably been in a deep trance throughout. In this state you will still be absorbing all the suggestions on an unconscious level. If you don't hear me counting at the end, you have probably drifted off to sleep at some point. In this case, you will absorb the suggestions only up to the point where you went to sleep. If this happens repeatedly, avoid listening when you are tired.

Initially I suggest that you listen to the recording on a daily basis. Once you feel you are in control, feel free to use it to reinforce all that you have learned at any time. There are no hard and fast rules as to how long you should use the audio for, as it will work differently for each individual. After listening a few times you should begin to notice some positive changes. Sometimes these changes will be instant and dramatic, or you may experience a gradual, subtle progression into new patterns of behaviour.

When you have listened to the relevant tracks enough times you will have acquired a deep-rooted belief that you *love* exercising, eating and sleeping well, and maintaining a level of fitness and positive attitude in your relationships, your career and your inner self will become effortless. Towards the end you will be instructed to repeat special hypnotic affirmations to help you to endorse your new healthy lifestyle. Belief plays a big part in re-programming. When you repeat these affirmations, say them with conviction and truly believe they are a reality. The stronger the feelings you create, the more effectively the affirmations will anchor themselves in your unconscious mind. So put your heart and soul into embracing your positive new beliefs.

As well as utilizing your feelings and emotions, the other main key to absorbing hypnotic suggestion is something called 'compounding'. This means that the more you hear the suggestions on the audio, along with the use of the self-hypnosis techniques, the quicker your unconscious mind will get the message. You will then respond to the suggestions automatically in your everyday life.

You will also hear a number of background affirmations echoed on both audio tracks, which will pan from left to right. This powerful method of delivering multiple suggestions simultaneously to the unconscious mind can help facilitate positive changes even more speedily. At the end of each recording you will be gently brought back to full waking consciousness with a mellow combination of suggestion and music. Finally, a series of positive subliminal suggestions embedded in the fade-out music is designed to facilitate the overall effect. These suggestions will reinforce the affirmation phrases printed in the book. Above all, remember that these techniques offer a broad brush approach and many can be adapted to suit your own requirements.

We are each blessed with the ability to imagine and when we learn how to harness that power we can achieve practically anything. Using your imagination as such a tool can help you make positive changes to the way you live your life. I sometimes liken the process to planting seeds in the fertile soil of your mind that, with love and attention, will grow into beautiful flowers. It is also a question of choice. You have the choice right now to make major changes to the way you live and to stop bad conditioning and events from your past jeopardizing your future health and happiness. Ultimately, the power of choice will help you draw on your own strengths and create an incredible self-belief that will enable you to live the rest of your life the way you have always wanted to live it.

Step 1

Healthy eating and hydration

'They say that age is all in your mind.
The trick is keeping it from creeping down into
your body.'

Author Unknown

Key Steps

Who among us doesn't look at old photographs of
ourselves and wonder what happened to the person
with smooth skin, who had so much energy, or was able
to slip into clothes several sizes smaller? And when we
think ahead to how many years we have left, we can't
help but wonder what the future might hold. Living
longer and looking younger have to be the ultimate
goals for all of us.

The good news is that, with the right help, it is easy

to turn back the clock and reset it to give you more time. There are four cornerstones for creating good health, increasing life expectancy, and achieving optimum vitality. They are:

- **diet**
- **exercise**
- **sleep**
- **a positive mental outlook**

Get those four elements right and you are well on the way to living longer and looking younger. Better still, you'll feel great about yourself, increase your self-confidence and be able to look to the future full of optimism. I will guide you through the process of achieving these goals. Forget the old dread of diets and exercise programmes you may have experienced in the past; say goodbye to sleepless nights and exhausted days feeling miserable or trying to catch up. With my help, you will be far better equipped to cope with these challenges than at any time in your life. Using my seven steps, you will develop the courage and self-belief to live life to the full. You will also learn to let go of your self-doubts and fears so that you can express your true potential. Together, we will take the first steps to a new, improved you – the first of which is maintaining a healthy diet.

You are not on this Earth to develop an overweight, sluggish body that devours sugar, fat and other harmful substances at an alarming rate, thereby dramatically cropping your life expectancy. In these days of fast food, trans-fats and binge drinking it is absolutely essential to be more mindful of what you eat and avoid harmful foods and drink that conspire against creating a healthy body. 'Eat to live, not live to eat' is a widely used ancient phrase because it is true.

Your power of choice

'Destiny is no matter of chance. It is a matter of choice: It is not a thing to be waited for; it is a thing to be achieved.'

William Jennings Bryan

There are many other reasons why people develop bad eating habits, but the thing to remember is that, regardless of what you may have done before, you have the power of choice. You can choose right now, this minute, to make changes to the way you eat and exercise. You no longer need to let poor conditioning or sloppy habits control your life; besides, it simply doesn't make sense to allow mistakes from your past to mess up your future. The techniques in this book and on the audio will help you overcome negative conditioning. They will allow you to move forward with a clean slate, and learn to believe that you deserve to be fit, healthy and in good shape.

Say that to yourself now:

I deserve to be fit and healthy and in good shape

If it feels good when you say it, then that's great. If affirming this phrase feels strange or uncomfortable at this stage, don't worry – by the end of the book and after using the audio download you will not only be saying it and believing it, but feeling good about it when you do.

Setting your weight goal

'It is for us to pray not for tasks equal to our powers, but for powers equal to our tasks; to go forward with a great desire forever beating at the door of our hearts as we travel toward our distant goal.'

Helen Keller

If you are overweight you need to set yourself a goal to achieve your optimum healthy weight. What should that be? There are all sorts of medical guidelines to help you decide, such as the BMI or body mass index, which is calculated by dividing your weight in kilograms by your height in metres squared to come up with a figure that – according to doctors – should be between 18.5 and 25. This figure has been calculated to show the weight for your height at which you are less likely to suffer from heart disease, cancer, diabetes and the myriad other health issues that go hand in hand with being overweight.

If you aren't sure what the healthiest weight is for your height, ask someone at your doctor's surgery to work it out for you, or check out the BMI calculators on the NHS Direct website. Remember that the BMI it gives you may be slightly misleading if you are over sixty, have a long-term medical condition, or are a weight-trainer or athlete carrying extra muscle. Also, the older you are, the more careful you have to be not to become too thin, or the process of slowing the speed at which you age could be hampered by the appearance of lines and wrinkles previously filled out by Nature's Botox – fat. Once you have decided on your ideal target weight, based on the levels that feel comfortable or healthy to you, then think carefully about it and don't set limits on that goal. Even if you weigh three hundred pounds (approximately twenty-one stone) or more, it is entirely possible for you to halve that in time. Take a moment now to decide on your ideal target weight for maximum health and longevity, and write it down:

My ideal target weight is _____

Once you have a clear goal in mind, I want you focus on a date by which you will reach that target. Be realistic, as losing weight too quickly can be counter-productive. Most diets fail because of one simple fact: your mind needs to adjust to your new self-image. So if you lose a lot of weight too speedily, your mind cannot adjust to your physical changes and may not recognize your new image because it hasn't caught up. This can create conflict and have a detrimental long-term effect, resulting in weight fluctuations and a failure to reach and maintain a healthy weight. For a lasting result, the best and most natural way to lose weight is slowly and steadily.

If, for example, you are one-hundred-and-seventy pounds (approximately twelve stone) now and your target weight is one-hundred-and-forty pounds (ten stone), allow yourself a comfortable six months to achieve this target. If you have a more ambitious target – for example to go from two-hundred-and-fifty pounds (or seventeen-and-a-half stone) to one hundred and fifty pounds (approximately ten-and-a-half stone) – then allow eighteen months to two years to achieve this, as you are looking to shed a third of your body weight and will need to take care. The message is not to rush; think of this as a long-term holistic journey in which you are empowering your mind and body more and more every day.

When you have decided upon both your ideal target weight and the time frame in which you will achieve this, I want you to write it down. This is a key step so please don't overlook it. Spend a few minutes now on setting a realistic goal. Write below: On (future date), I will weigh (your ideal target weight):

On _____

I will weigh _____

Write this goal down on several different pieces of paper and put them where you will read them every day. On your bedside table perhaps, on the fridge door, the dashboard of your car or stuck to your bathroom mirror, because you need to see your goal regularly. You can even set your weight goal and date as a frequent reminder on your mobile phone or computer, or stick it up somewhere in your workspace. The more you see your goal and read the promise you have made yourself, the better. Seeing these targets every day is vital as this reinforces your determination and desire to achieve them every time you read them. It is crucial to stay focused.

For this reason, it is also better to avoid discussing your goals. If anyone notices that you've lost weight or wants to know how you are achieving it, just tell them you are creating a healthier lifestyle for yourself. This is your body, your programme, and your business. Nobody else's. However well-intentioned, others will always be full of advice and opinions that may introduce negative energy, self-doubt, or make you wonder if you should try it their way instead. You need to keep true to yourself and what we are doing together. To stay focused, it is vital that you take personal responsibility for yourself, and do not ask others to help you or influence you in a way that may divert you from your path.

Each of these small steps will add up to a powerful and lasting solution which will give you total control of your weight like never before. It will completely take the struggle out of the equation. After using the audio and self-hypnosis techniques, your habits will start to change. You may find yourself automatically turning down the offer of something you would have previously accepted like chocolate or cake, or you may feel an inner pull driving you to take up an activity like tennis or running.

As you begin to add all of the small steps and techniques together, I guarantee you things will change easily and effortlessly. Once you create your own programme that confirms you are a fit and healthy person, this is exactly what you will become.

Using your creative mind

'Age is an issue of mind over matter.
If you don't mind, it doesn't matter.'

Mark Twain

Visual imagery is a powerful way of absorbing beliefs into your unconscious mind. By seeing yourself as you want yourself to be one day – slim, fit and healthy, enjoying life to the full with friends and family – you will be able to keep to your targets more easily. A key ingredient in re-programming is that the mind doesn't distinguish between what is real and what is imagined so that when you create a visualization your mind will accept it as a reality. Regular visualization will help you to remain focused and gradually alter your perception of your self-image, which will make future habit changes easier. Be creative and make your visualizations colourful and elaborate, with as much detail as possible. Immerse yourself *totally* in the visualizations and use all of your senses to make them realistic. Most importantly, invest your feelings strongly into them.

When, in your mind's eye, you see yourself at your target weight looking and feeling great, go into detail and notice all the things that have changed for the better now you are at this new weight. Run images in your mental cinema like a short film, adding as much information as possible. For instance, if your goal is to be a certain weight, shape and size for a wedding or party in six months time, see yourself at this event, wearing a great new outfit, looking fantastic and receiving praise from your fellow guests. Imagine yourself having a wonderful, happy time. Feel your beautiful clothes against your skin and take note of how good they feel. Make the whole picture bright and clear and use as many of your senses as you can. Most importantly, always see yourself in a completely positive light, looking fabulous and feeling in control, while expressing yourself clearly and confidently.

You can use visualization techniques to prepare yourself for events such as an exam, a sporting challenge, public speaking, business or social occasions. There is no need to blow a great new opportunity through nerves or anxiety. Learning these techniques can help anyone overcome anxiety in pressure situations. Footballers, golfers and others sportspeople regularly use visualization to prepare themselves mentally before a competition. Businesspeople, too, find it an effective tool prior to important meetings or conferences. By seeing themselves winning, delivering a great speech or making a successful presentation, they are able to condition their brains into believing that they can do so.

More amazing still, and as I mentioned in my introduction, studies have proven that just by visualizing exercise your body will respond and show signs of increased conditioning. The breakthrough study at the Cleveland Clinic Foundation in Ohio split thirty healthy young people into three groups and had them think about different things. The first had to visualize moving their little fingers, the second group had to imagine exercising their bicep muscles, and the third – the control group – were not asked to undertake any visualization at all. Researchers found that the volunteers in the first group increased the strength in their little fingers by more than thirteen per cent, in the second they increased their bicep strength by an incredible fifty-three per cent. The control group showed no increase in muscle strength at all. Furthermore, the gains lasted for three months after they had stopped their mental exercise regime. (Source: *From mental power to muscle power: gaining strength by using the mind*, Vinoth K. Ranganathan, Vlodek Siemionowa, Jing Z. Liu, Vinod Sahgal, and Guang H. Yue, *Neuropsychologia 42* (2004) 944–956)

The possible repercussions of this research are endless. Victims of accidents, strokes or sports injuries could, in theory, be trained to visualize themselves better, maybe even be coached into rebuilding neural pathways in the brain or repairing damaged nerves and tissues. Imagine that. Simply by harnessing the power of the mind, you can actually change your life, which is why losing weight and adopting a healthier lifestyle using self-hypnosis is so easy.

The following technique is a good starting point in learning to programme your brain with positive thoughts and familiarizing yourself with a gentle trance state. You can build this technique into your daily routines at any time, revisiting this script and developing a strong intention so that your mind has a clear image of your ideal weight, shape and size. Read the script through until you know what to do, and then practise this visualization every day ideally for three weeks. After that, you can refresh it every now and again. As with all things, practice makes perfect and you will find that the more you practise the deeper you will go and the more realistic your visualization will become. You can spend as little as ten minutes creating the images and feelings that work for you or you can spend much longer if you prefer. The important thing is repeating the visualization each day so that you strengthen your new mental programme.

The future visualization technique

Find a quiet room with no distractions. Get comfortable, close your eyes and focus on your breathing, inhaling slowly through your nose and out through your mouth, feeling your ribcage expanding as you do so. Breathe away any tension in your body with each out-breath and gradually allow yourself to relax. As you do so, clear away any unwanted thoughts until your mind is still and quiet. Focus on the stillness of the moment.

Now imagine going forward in time to the date you have set to reach your target weight. Stay relaxed and focus on this simple thought. Now visualize yourself at your target weight looking slimmer, fitter and healthier. Amplify the positive feelings and make the image big, bright and clear. See yourself standing in front of a full-length mirror, dressed in a favourite outfit, looking great and feeling attractive and confident with your new shape and size. Use all of your senses to make it real. Feel your clothes; smile back at your own reflection. Run your hands down your slim physique and praise yourself as you do so. Now accept on every level that this is what you deserve. Hold this picture in your mind and affirm to yourself silently or out loud: 'I love being fit and healthy. I love being in control of my weight.' Accept that you have lost any need or desire for unhealthy, fattening food, and take a moment to relish your positive feelings about the new you. These feelings and images will sink into your unconscious mind and become a part of your inner reality, helping you work towards your goal with ease.

When you are ready, allow your mind to clear, slowly count to ten, open your eyes, and come back to full waking consciousness. When you reach the number ten every part of you will be back in the here and now. Remember to practise this visualization often, especially at the beginning of your journey.

Detoxification

> 'Time may be a great healer, but it's a lousy beautician.'
>
> *Author Unknown*

If you want to break free of your addictions to caffeine, sugar, cigarettes, chocolate, alcohol or anything unhealthy, then a detoxifying programme is an excellent place to start. This usually involves spending a week or more on a diet of fruit, vegetables and nuts, drinking only water or herbal tea, thereby cutting out the poisons and toxins that have been clogging your body for so long. Some of you may recoil in horror at the thought of such abstinence, but I can assure you it is a fantastic experience and something that reaps huge benefits, and quickly. With the right mental approach, you can learn to love the process and even look forward to the next time, anticipating how good it will make you feel.

An increasing number of people choose to give up alcohol for the month of January, keen to purge themselves of the excesses of Christmas and New Year. A fuller detox programme is one step further on from this, and will give your body a chance to repair and recover itself. As a way of kick-starting your new programme of improved health and vitality, there is nothing to beat it.

My first experience of detoxing was when I went to a yoga and meditation retreat in a remote part of southern Turkey. I wasn't particularly unfit at the time but was keen to improve my levels of fitness. For the first three days, we ate nothing solid and drank only specially prepared fruit and vegetable smoothies, three times a day. This may sound austere but when you are in a positive environment with thirty other people from all walks of life sharing the experience with you, it is surprisingly easy to do; especially when the juices were not only delicious but meticulously blended to give us all the vitamins and minerals our bodies needed.

After a week of detoxing, plus practising meditation, yoga and swimming, I felt amazing and had more energy than I'd enjoyed in years. I lost weight and my fitness levels increased dramatically. Between us, our group collectively lost one-hundred-and-fifty pounds – the weight of one person. On our last day, my wife at the time was amused to overhear me chatting to fellow guests on how clear and sparkling their eyes were. I was amazed to see how healthy everyone looked after just one week of taking good care of themselves. If I hadn't realized it before, the fact that eating healthily makes you feel great was massively reinforced. And by removing yourself from everyday foods for a while, you quickly come to realize that so much of the processed and packaged food we eat – even the stuff labelled 'low fat', 'sugar free' or 'healthy' – is full of refined sugars, salts and additives that are bad for us and slow us down. Healthy, organic food has exactly the opposite effect.

You don't have to travel to Turkey to experience what I did. You can detox at home for a week or more to cleanse your system and break free of any destructive eating habits. A strict detox is not recommended over a long period, but in short bursts it is an excellent way of freeing yourself from addictions. If I had any weight to lose, I would immediately start with a one- or two-week detox to purge my body and prepare it for a healthier regime. That's all it takes – a couple of weeks of your time to set you on your new path. Do it in the comfort of your own home in a period when there are few demands on your time and energy. Take advice from an expert or read a book on the subject to make sure you are giving yourself enough nutrients and vitamins. You should also do some gentle exercise each day, although nothing too strenuous. Check with your doctor if you are at all unsure.

Buy a juicer if you haven't already got one and whiz through a combination of delicious fruit and vegetables to create high-energy drinks. After a few trips to the greengrocers to stock up on organic produce, you will start to feel really good about taking control of your eating and helping yourself to better health. This, in turn, will inspire you to live ever more healthily. The first few days on a detox may give you the occasional headache or even make you feel rough as you wean yourself off the unhealthy products your body has come to depend on, but this is simply because it is letting go of toxins, not because the process is bad for you. After three days you will start to feel much better and, if you are exercising as well, you will notice your energy rising. After one week you will feel amazing – full of energy, a few pounds lighter, and your eyes will sparkle like a film star's.

There are many detox programmes you can buy that come with pre-prepared powders and vitamin supplements. These are said to stimulate digestion, activate glands in the intestines, and increase bile and urine elimination. Toxins are expelled in a mild and natural way through the kidneys, liver and intestines. This process in turn will help to renew and rejuvenate your body and mind. Never underestimate the effect food has on your mood and brainpower.

The main benefits you will experience will include improved sleep, increased energy levels, and softer features as ageing lines and wrinkles smooth out with the combination of rehydration and a purer food intake. You may also find that minor ailments will disappear. There are so many other bonuses – such as watching your body change its shape and your skin begin to glow – that the experience will change you forever and motivate you to make your health and well-being a priority. What could be more important, after all? If you want to change your life, then start now. Once you do, you will enjoy the discovery that eating food that benefits your body is so much better than gorging on sickly, fattening or processed food that leaves you lethargic, bloated and full of guilt. Once you follow this healthy path you will feel so glad that you did. Your only regret will be not having done it sooner!

Detoxing case study

Sarah was not in the best of health when she came to work for me a few years ago. An overweight wife and mother, having accumulated several bad lifestyle habits by the age of thirty-eight, she longed to get back to the slender, energetic young woman she had once been. With my help, and inspired by my many clients and testimonials from satisfied customers, she began a detox and diet programme that worked for her.

Within just three months, she had lost three stone and remains fit and healthy to this day. At her fortieth birthday party she looked and felt fabulous, having focused on that as her goal. 'I honestly never thought I'd manage it,' she admitted afterwards. 'Secretly, I was resigned to being overweight and unhealthy, thinking it was too late for me. But if I can do it, anyone can. The hypnosis recording and sessions helped me realize that I could achieve my goals. If you really put your mind to something, you can do it. I am the proof!'

Hydration

'We turn not older with years, but newer every day.'

Emily Dickinson

You are going to learn techniques to help you *unlearn* bad habits from the past. Just as it is now widely accepted that it is good to clean and floss your teeth regularly, for example, or to wear a seat belt when driving, so you will acquire new beliefs to create good habits.

Water is the most precious commodity on this Earth. It makes up more than sixty per cent of the human body and seventy per cent of the human brain. Without water, we would die and our planet would not survive. Think of a plant that hasn't been watered recently; how it curls and wrinkles, losing all its colour and vibrancy. With one top-up from a watering can, the plant will quickly flourish and thrive again, growing tall, its flowers vibrant and attractive. Use that visualization to imagine the effects of water on your body, your skin and your vitality.

Once you get into the habit of drinking lots of water at regular intervals throughout the day – and ideally you should aim to get your levels up to four litres of filtered or mineral water a day – you will start to notice instant benefits. Water flushes away toxins, cleanses the kidneys, improves complexion, aids digestion and helps fill you up so that you don't feel the need to snack between meals.

Many people don't drink enough water and are constantly dehydrated. Various studies have shown that – apart from the beneficial effects on skin, eyes and hair – dehydration can lead to depression, anxiety and sleep deprivation. A recent study at an old people's home in Suffolk, England, found that by encouraging residents to drink at least eight glasses of water every day, staff reduced the number of falls dramatically and found that the residents were more alert and less confused. Nurses at a hospital in Buckinghamshire recorded a forty-five per cent drop in hospital admissions by care home residents after piloting a similar scheme. A well-named 'Thirst 4 Life' initiative has been adopted in several areas, as part of a national scheme called Water for Health Alliance. Official NHS guidelines state: *'Encouraging people to drink enough water in their diet and to stay hydrated can make an important contribution to illness prevention, and directly supports the health of our population.'*

The British Dental Health Foundation asserts: *'Water, along with milk, is the only drink that the Foundation recommends as completely safe for teeth. It contains no sugar, no calories and no acid and, from a holistic point of view, by guarding against everything from headaches to heart disease it is massively important to a person's overall health.'*

The following technique should help you learn to love the taste of water. It works on a deeper level to create new beliefs that you will respond to automatically.

The love water technique

Close your eyes and take a few slow deep breaths. Centre your mind and repeat the following affirmation to yourself over and over, in a slow rhythmic chant: 'I love the taste of pure fresh water.' As you affirm this, visualize crystal-clear water pouring into your mouth – refreshing, tingling, cleansing. Taste the water on your tongue and really enjoy the sensation of drinking it, as it soothes your throat and fills you with purity. When you have opened your eyes, drink a large glass of bottle or filtered water and notice how good it tastes. Keep using this visualization and before long, you will be well on the way to creating a healthy habit that will last a lifetime.

Nutrition

'Anyone who stops learning is old, whether at twenty or eighty.'

Henry Ford

Everyone wants a quick solution to feeling more energetic, slimmer and fitter. Having an internal spring-clean through a detoxification programme is all well and good but if you then go back to the way you were before, you won't achieve any long-term results. Lifestyle changes are needed and you must become aware of what you are putting into your mouth, how much you are eating or drinking and where it's coming from. By this I mean how fresh it is, whether it is from a packet or tin, is laden with sugar or salt, or if it is blasted in a microwave until there is no life force left in it.

One in three people now gets cancer and the same percentage develops diabetes. These diseases have reached epic proportions largely because people don't take good enough care of themselves and regularly eat food loaded with toxins. Such chemicals are the major source of high toxic levels in the body, since most processed food nowadays is pumped full of additives in the quest for maximum shelf life at the cheapest possible price. The food industry is worth billions of dollars and in such a highly competitive and commercial world, businesses have one aim – to maximise their profits. This means that people unwittingly consume food packed with chemicals every day; chemicals that combine with those already polluting our air and water to overload the body and make it toxic and vulnerable to disease.

Once you start to make informed decisions about the food and drink you consume, you will feel better and more in control. After years of bad habits, we tend to do a lot of things automatically, but stopping and thinking about what it is that we are doing can be life-changing. If you keep a diary of what you eat in an average week, for example, you might realize that you're actually consuming too many bars of chocolate or too many cups of coffee, drinking too many units of alcohol to be healthy or skipping meals and eating at the wrong time of day. A recent study found that those that kept a food diary lost far more weight than those who didn't.

As well as drinking four litres of water daily, begin each day with hot water and a slice of fresh lemon or lime. Substitute a fresh fruit juice or smoothie for your usual breakfast cereal or toast. Cut down on bread, biscuits and cakes, and avoid snacking between meals. If you are hungry, have a piece of fruit or some nuts instead. Eat three balanced meals a day and include plenty of fresh vegetables. Ensure at least one meal contains a large leafy green salad. Raw vegetables are wonderful for helping your body cleanse itself and the bulk they create helps fill you up more quickly.

Consulting a nutritionist or naturopath might be worthwhile. However, there are many simple changes, like the ones mentioned above, that you can start to make yourself and which will help you onto the right track. Go to your local library or bookshop and read up on the subject. See what your health food shop has in terms of general nutritional advice. Ask your GP for what help your surgery may offer. Eating healthily doesn't mean short-changing yourself or feeling hungry all the time. With the right ingredients you can fill yourself up with delicious, nutritious food that will soon give you fantastic results – a renewed and rejuvenated self. Once you acquire your new good habits, they soon become conditioned into your daily life to permanently improve your diet and health.

The main thing I have learned from more than twenty years of being a hypnotherapist is that the mind has unlimited potential. It is fear that stops us living life to the full, and fear of *change* that prevents us moving forward. Use the following technique to harness the unlimited power of your mind to live the way you know is best for you – free of the unhealthy foods that have been holding you back.

Slow food case study

I recently worked with thirty-six-year-old Alison who was at least two stone overweight when she first came to see me. She had tried many diets in the past, all of which had failed. Seeing a hypnotherapist was her last resort. I explained that this is a new holistic approach and that she should forget the word 'diet' altogether. What she needed to do was simply change her patterns of behaviour and re-programme her mind to accept them. One of the first things I asked her to visualize under hypnosis was to make a habit of eating slowly and to be consciously aware of each mouthful she ate.

Alison worked on this goal as well as regularly visualizing her weight goal. She detoxed, drank more water and within a short time had achieved her weight goal of nine-and-a-half stone. For the first time ever she is maintaining this weight with ease, as her new healthy approach to food is firmly entrenched in her conscious and unconscious routines.

Banishing unhealthy food technique

Close your eyes and take a few slow, deep breaths. Allow your mind to clear. Take a moment to go inside yourself and totally relax. When you are ready, imagine a plate piled high with rotting fish riddled with maggots, or something similarly putrid that is absolutely repulsive to you. Create this picture in your mind's eye and connect with the revolting smell of the fish. Don't gag but make this image and smell truly real. Take a moment to do this.

Once you have a clear picture and can almost see the maggots wriggling or sense the stench in your nostrils, bring to mind the one unhealthy item of food that you want to erase from your diet and mix it with the rotting fish. If it is chocolate, imagine the chocolate melting all over the fish, sticking to the fins and slimy scales. If it is crisps, think of them going soggy as they soak up the leaking bodily fluids of the rotting fish. If your weakness is a fizzy drink, imagine one of the dead fish bobbing up and down inside a glass of pop, its milky eye glinting at you through the bubbles.

Be creative with this part of the technique; the

more vivid you can make this image, the more powerful it will be. Allow a few minutes to digest this disgusting image and odour, and then let your mind go blank. Take a few slow breaths, slowly count to three and open your eyes. The next time you think about the food or drink that you mixed up with the rotting fish you will feel completely different. You will have lost any desire for that food or drink, or you may even find it repulsive.

You can use this technique to systematically eradicate all bad foods and drinks from your diet. Focus on eliminating one thing at a time and make sure you have lost all desire for it before moving on to the next.

You are going to build a powerful and lasting inner desire to lose weight and become fit and healthy. Easily. You are not going to discuss your plan with anyone or try to impress others when you do begin to lose weight. This journey is for you and you alone. You are going to remain disciplined and focused. You have chosen to embark on a holistic weight loss programme to improve the quality of your life, so you must be totally honest with yourself.

You are your own best therapist. Only you can break the negative patterns of the past. Breaking free of unwanted habits is easy with hypnosis. Together, we will re-programme your mind to come up with an eating and rehydration plan which is perfect for you. You have nothing to lose and everything to gain. So what is stopping you? Only your own inaction. No more excuses. Make the decision now to take positive action towards a new healthier, happier you.

Golden rule 1
healthy eating

• Get into the habit of eating slowly and chewing your food for much longer. This should be a golden rule from now on and something you cultivate consciously. Eating slowly and chewing your food well serves to satisfy your taste buds more completely, enabling you to feel satiated quickly. Importantly, it also helps your body to digest the food more easily. You must adopt this habit whenever you eat. And remember, as soon as you feel full, stop eating, even if there is food left on your plate. If you were ever taught that you must always clear your plate, that old conditioning no longer applies to you now.

• Cut down or eradicate all junk food and drink from your diet such as any processed food, tinned food, white flour products, sugar products, caffeine, chocolate, cola and fizzy sugar drinks in general, alcohol, fatty foods, fried foods, foods containing additives. Minimize your salt intake.

- Buy a juicer and blender and get in the habit of making fresh juices or smoothies every day. Begin each day with a freshly prepared juice and – if the opportunity allows – have more during the day. Juicing regularly is a key element in the process of health and longevity.

- If this rule seems a stretch, then follow the 80/20 rule. If eighty per cent of the time you are eating the right healthy food you can afford the odd indulgence twenty per cent of the time. However, if you do occasionally indulge in chocolate or wine for example, make sure they are organic brands of the highest quality.

Step 2

Exercise and fitness

'There are people whose watch stops at a certain hour and who remain permanently at that age.'

Charles Augustin Sainte-Beuve

General maintenance

If you owned a car you were especially fond of, you wouldn't fill it with low-quality fuel or fail to maintain it. You would look after it, and figure out how best to optimize its performance. You would take it for regular services and – the minute something went wrong – you'd whip it straight into a garage and ask an expert to help you fix it.

Why is it that we often take better care of our material possessions than we do of our own bodies? Well-maintained, the body is a magnificent feat of engineering. It will run perfectly if you give it the right fuel and keep it in good condition. Just recently, there was a story in the newspapers of a man who had owned the same 1939 Austin for almost fifty years, loving it and looking after it so that, even after three hundred thousand miles on the clock, it was still running perfectly, gleamed as if brand new, and had never caused him any trouble. Looking at a photograph of this stoic octogenarian who was still driving regularly and enjoying life to the full, I suspected he treated his own body just as carefully.

Now that you have learned about the best fuels with which to feed your engine, the next step is to improve the condition of your bodywork. There is one sure way of doing this and achieving results quickly and enjoyably – exercise. Regular physical activity has numerous benefits, not least that it will help slow down the ageing process as you become lithe, supple and increasingly full of energy. Better still, endorphins – known as the 'happy hormones' or 'feel-good chemicals' in your brain – are released when you exercise and help to clear away negative emotions to improve the mood. So you're not only doing yourself good, you'll feel good about it too.

Exercise increases blood flow to the brain and body, stimulates the nervous system and triggers the release of adrenaline, which has an uplifting effect. It helps lower blood pressure, improves circulation to expel toxins, increases the metabolic rate to better fight disease and burn fat, and releases physical stress and tension in the body by loosening the muscles. For those facing the possibility of osteoporosis or brittle bone disease in old age, repeated resistance exercises like aerobics, trampolining, using weights, running or even just walking can dramatically strengthen the bones and the muscles that support them. In short, exercise has both a serious effect on life expectancy and on quality of life. All in all, it's a no-brainer. When it is included as part of a holistic approach, along with changes to diet and lifestyle, it can be one of the most important weapons in the fight against ill health, ageing and anxiety.

Make a plan

'Health is the vital principle of bliss, and exercise, of health.'

James Thomson

Each and every day, look for as many ways as possible in which you can become more active and mobile. This can be something as simple as using the stairs at work instead of the lift, or walking or cycling to the shops rather than driving. Simply moving about and being more active will help you burn calories. Most of the excuses people make for being overweight are myths, like claiming to be 'big-boned' or having a slow metabolism. If you eat healthily and exercise regularly, you lose weight and become fit. It is a simple as that. Your personal metabolic rate is not something you are born or stuck with; it is something you can control. If you sit in front of the television every night, eating crisps and never exercising, you will develop a slow metabolism. When you become more active and exercise often, your metabolic rate will speed up and you will lose weight more easily. It's up to you. The desire for change has to come from within. You have the power to choose.

To achieve this healthy level of physical fitness and become more active, you need to seize every opportunity to do so. For example, if you can't park right outside a restaurant, house or shop you're visiting, don't get frustrated; park a few hundred metres away and walk. Use the inconvenience as an opportunity to get a little exercise. Having a short stroll after leaving a restaurant will help you to digest your meal and burn a few calories. When you go to the supermarket, get into the habit of parking your car in a space furthest from the entrance not closest to it. Walk briskly to the bus stop or railway station beyond the one you normally use. As you begin to incorporate these ideas into your daily life, they soon become habits that you'll learn to accept and enjoy. They cost little time and become part of your everyday approach to your fitness. There is always another way of viewing things and, if you reframe your attitude towards exercise, you will never again be disappointed because an elevator isn't working or because you can't find a parking space.

Many people make a bold decision to get fit, only to give up a few months later and drift back to their old unhealthy ways. It is a fact that fitness clubs oversell their memberships because eighty per cent of those who join stop going after three months. If everyone turned up at once they wouldn't be able to cope! To improve your fitness levels in the longer term, you must adopt a mindset that says you are creating a new, holistic, healthy lifestyle. Think of the fable of the tortoise and the hare, in which the slow but steady pace of the tortoise brought success while the hare burned itself out. Use this story as your metaphor for your long-term goal. Work on your fitness slowly by doing a little each day and building up to a level that feels good for you.

It may help to find new hobbies and pastimes that fit in with your new healthy lifestyle. I highly recommend yoga, Pilates or a similar discipline as part of a holistic approach to achieving a weight loss goal. Yoga, especially, is a fantastic discipline for toning the body and focusing the mind. The best way to learn is in a class, but if you don't have time to join one there are many good DVDs and videos available online. The beauty of yoga is that once you learn the basics, you can create your own version of a programme and focus on toning specific parts of the body. If yoga doesn't appeal, then find a different healthy pursuit that you enjoy and that you can do regularly to increase your metabolic rate. Swimming, tennis and badminton offer good aerobic exercise and are enjoyable too. Aim to do some form of exercise every day, even if it is a short, brisk walk or a ten-minute bounce on a mini-trampoline. This is a great way to start the day and I can't recommend it highly enough for a daily exercise that you will grow to love.

When creating an exercise programme that works for you and that you can incorporate into your day, factor in that the ideal time for this is first thing in the morning – before your breakfast juice. The more you practise, the stronger your desire to further increase your fitness will become. You don't need any apparatus, but if you feel like it go out and buy some weights, a mini-trampoline or an exercise ball. Failing that, work out your own routine incorporating sit-ups, stretching, or using household items as weights (always make sure you take proper advice first).

If you follow these steps for twenty-one days, then that is all it will take for these routines to become something you'll want to do forever. Little and often is the key.

Key steps

The key steps to starting a new fitness programme are:

- Avoid junk food or drinks.

- Stick to three main meals and drink lots of fresh water throughout each day.

- Make yourself fresh juices or smoothies at least once a day. Use a variety of fruit and vegetables, preferably organic.

- Start with a ten-minute work-out each morning, or find another activity that you love and do it daily.

- Be as active as possible in your daily life, seizing every opportunity to move your body.

- Empower your mind by using self-hypnosis and/or listening to the audio download every day.

Fitness case study

Jim, a fifty-six-year-old engineer, came to me having recently been diagnosed with type 2 diabetes and chest problems. He was overweight and unfit and had picked up a lot of unhealthy habits in the previous twenty years. He hoped that I could just hypnotize him and all his weight would drop off within a short period of time. When I quizzed him about his younger life, he revealed that he had once been a champion squash player, a game he believed he would never play again. Under hypnosis, I suggested to Jim that he might want to resume his interest in squash – gently at first and only under the supervision of his doctor – combining his new fitness regime with some healthy eating choices. Six months later, Jim wrote to thank me for my help. He had lost two stone, was playing squash twice a week and – better still – was no longer at risk from long-term diabetes. He said the whole process has been almost effortless with the help of hypnosis and my audio recording, and that his life had been transformed. He sent me a photograph of him in his sports kit and I barely recognized the athletic man in the picture who looked ten years younger than when he had walked – wheezily – into my office.

Smoking

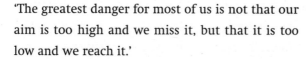

'The greatest danger for most of us is not that our
aim is too high and we miss it, but that it is too
low and we reach it.'

Michelangelo

If you don't smoke or have recently given up, then well
done, you won't have to read this section. If you do
smoke, however, or are still in the process of giving up
and worry that you could slip back into your old habits
at any time, then this demands your fullest attention.

The dangers of smoking to general health are so well
known and so heavily plastered in dire warnings all
over the packets that they are not necessary to repeat
here. You would have had to have been a hermit not to
know that even smoking a few cigarettes a day massively
raises the risk of dying of cancer and heart disease as
well as being linked to a host of other diseases including
diabetes. What may not be so widely known is how
closely smoking is also linked to premature ageing as
well as shortening of life. We all know that smokers
tend to be more heavily wrinkled, with greying, rough
skin and sallow features but recent research in Japan
has found out why. The study at Nagoya City University
Medical School found that smoking attacks the skin

cells and destroys their ability to regenerate themselves. Cells exposed to smoke produced a far greater quantity of the enzyme that is responsible for breaking down skin. This enzyme prevents the skin from constantly renewing itself or making replacement tissue, causing wrinkles and age lines. The researchers also found that smoke caused a drop in the production of fresh collagen – the secret to a youthful skin – by up to forty per cent.

Smoking also causes irreparable damage to teeth and gums, increasing bacteria in plaque, causing widespread discolouration, decay and loss – a key factor in adding years to a face. It affects eyes and hair as it depletes the levels of vitamin C in the body, and weakens the immune system and therefore its ability to fight infection. Add this to the serious risks to the major organs that threaten the entire balance and health of the body and it becomes clear that smoking – perhaps more than any other factor – is the chief culprit in the crime of premature ageing. If for no other reason than vanity, there has never been a better time to stop.

Just as you can retrain your mind to dislike fattening foods, sweets and unhealthy drinks and to genuinely love vegetables, fruit and water, so you can learn to dislike smoking. If you create a habit of consciously doing this, your mind will absorb and assimilate these affirmations and in time you will create a new healthy reality. You will soon find yourself reaching for a mineral water instead of a coffee or a piece of chewing gum instead of a cigarette *and* enjoying it.

Most people's first experience of smoking is an ordeal. Remember that first cigarette when you were a kid? You probably coughed and choked and spluttered and thought, 'This tastes horrible! What's all the fuss about?' But because you wanted to be grown up and smoke like an adult you trained yourself, through gritted teeth, to like it. The habit sticks and suddenly you find you can't do without cigarettes. Bizarre isn't it? I know because I was a smoker until I quit for good twenty years ago.

Many smokers even brainwash themselves into believing that cigarettes make them feel better and help them to relax. In truth, nicotine is a toxic nerve poison that constricts arteries and increases adrenaline production to raise blood pressure in order to overcome this constriction, thus stimulating the entire nervous system. People only relax with a cigarette because they have conditioned themselves to *believe* they will. You must rid yourself completely of that belief. You will now learn alternative ways to relax and feel composed without needing to rely on nicotine. For example, if I told you every time you gave your right ear lobe a gentle tug you would feel relaxed, after a while this would become a reality. Your unconscious mind unquestioningly believes what you tell it – especially when you compound a belief through repetition.

Smoking case study

One thing I realized early on is that the power of hypnosis is not always about the hypnotherapist. It is about the belief of the individual and how much they want their goal to happen. One of my earliest clients demonstrated this perfectly. He was very nervous about being hypnotized but was desperate to stop smoking. We discussed the common myths about hypnosis and I assured him that the experience would be nothing like the stage shows he'd seen. I explained that he would be in control at all times and that I was simply guiding him.

He relaxed but while we were discussing his passion for football he suddenly sat bolt upright and fixed his eyes on mine. He then began swaying from side to side and said, 'Ooh, you're doing it to me now!' He continued to sway, fully believing that I had started to hypnotize him, which I hadn't. He then went into the deepest trance I'd ever witnessed and I hadn't even begun the induction stage of my hypnotherapy session yet. Being relatively inexperienced at that time, I was bewildered.

Sticking to my training, I instructed him to lie down, and spent the next thirty minutes going through my script, which I later realized was largely unnecessary. He was already in an extremely receptive state and would have accepted suggestions easily at that point. I eventually guided him out of the trance, whereupon he announced he felt great and happily went on his way. I heard later from a family member that the man had remained a committed non-smoker ever since. It made me realize where the real power in hypnosis lies – with the individual and what they believe they can achieve. Belief is everything. Create the belief first and your reality will follow.

When you are eating well, exercising, cutting back on your drinking and not smoking, you must never think of any of it as a hardship or that you're losing something. Always focus on what it is giving you – your health. If you make a conscious habit of saying to yourself that you hate cigarettes, your mind will eventually get the message and you will indeed end up hating cigarettes. So why not programme your mind and make that choice right now? Think of it as a wonderful gift that you have this incredible mind that you can programme for your own good.

Once you decide you are going to stop smoking you must be absolutely clear in your own mind that you are breaking the habit forever. Set yourself a date to quit and then use my self-hypnosis technique every day. This will reinforce your goal on an unconscious level and help you to quit with ease. I gave up in 1989 after fifteen years of puffing away. Breaking free of that particular bad habit was one of the most satisfying things I've ever done. My only regret was that I hadn't done it sooner. The truth is that when you really want to stop smoking forever you simply do it. You no longer stop for a while and then try and find an excuse to start again. When you use the power of your mind to focus on the fact that you are a non-smoker it becomes a reality and you free yourself from the habit completely.

The following technique should help you in your own quest to improve your general health and well-being by giving up smoking. The stresses of addressing such a highly addictive and destructive habit can be halved with the use of hypnosis and many clients have success-fully quit with my help or by using my audio downloads.

Give up smoking now

Begin to breathe slowly and deeply in through your nose and out through your mouth with a steady rhythm. If you can, close your eyes to focus on your breathing. Visualize drawing pure fresh air into your lungs and clearing away any stale air with every out-breath. Enjoy the feeling of the clean air filling your lungs and continue breathing away any traces of stale air.

Continue this slow, rhythmical breathing and, as you inhale, push your stomach out so that you breathe into your stomach cavity, expanding it with your in-breath. As you exhale, let your stomach contract and your chest expand. Practise this breathing cycle for a while until it comes naturally. Once you have the hang of diaphragmatic breathing, make each in-breath last as long as possible so that you fill all of your lungs. Then, at the top of each breath hold it for three seconds – one, two, three. Exhale very slowly and count to five as you do so.

Continue with this pattern keeping your breathing slow and steady. You will soon begin to feel physically relaxed and mentally calm. In this state, allow your mind to go blank and slip deeper into relaxation. With your mind still and quiet, imagine you are now a non-smoker. See yourself in situations where previously you would have smoked but are now completely smoke free. Visualize yourself looking happy and content as a non-smoker, feeling and looking fitter and healthier. Amplify the positive feelings and make the image big, bright and clear. Use all of your senses to make it real. Now accept on every level that this is what you deserve. You deserve to be free of nicotine forever. You are a non-smoker. Hold this picture in your mind and affirm to yourself silently or out loud:

I love being free from smoking.
I remain a non-smoker forever.
I love being fit and healthy.
I find the taste and smell of nicotine repulsive.

Feel each statement as a reality as you affirm them. You can also add your own affirmations but make sure they are along the same lines. When you are ready to finish, allow your mind to clear for a minute, then count slowly upwards from one to ten. Open your eyes when you reach the number eight and at the number ten you will come back to full waking consciousness:

1 ... 2 ... 3 ... 4 ... 5 ... 6 ... 7 ... 8 ... 9 ... 10.

Repeat this technique daily until you are completely free of any desire to smoke. Any time you get an old smoking trigger use the diaphragmatic breathing exercise instead. One thing to be aware of when you quit is that your body is making a big adjustment so you need to give it as much help as possible in the early stages. I recommend you cut down on coffee, tea and alcohol as this will minimize your smoking triggers. It is also advisable to drink lots of water to help flush traces of nicotine and other toxins out of your system. Once the nicotine leaves your system completely sugar levels can drop which can sometimes cause an urge for nicotine. To balance this adjustment, get into the habit of eating two to three oranges or pink grapefruits a day. I also strongly recommend you take a vitamin B complex. The good news is that after four days the nicotine will have gone from your system. After ten days you'll begin to feel really good. Your lung capacity will be increased by up to a third, oxygen levels in your bloods cells will be back to normal and all the residual poisons will be completely cleansed from your body. After a month your circulation will improve and energy levels increase. Each day that passes as a non-smoker your chance of heart or lung disease dramatically decreases.

Hypnosis and health

'Thou should eat to live, not live to eat.'

Socrates

My ex-wife Aly and I went on a cruise once. We had never been on one before and thought it might be a nice thing to do. It was, and we enjoyed our vacation. But one of the things that amazed us most about the experience was the unedifying spectacle of people massively over-indulging and gorging themselves. You know the type – those that go to 'all you can eat' buffets and return time and again, their plates laden with enough food to feed at least two people. On a cruise, all the food and drink is inclusive so – to get their 'money's worth' – people often feel they have to gobble up every mouthful, especially at the enormous self-service midnight buffet served just a few hours after dinner.

Everyone likes to enjoy themselves and not worry about what they're eating and drinking on holiday – me included. But there has to be a point at which a light bulb comes on in the brain and flashes the message that, when you have already eaten three full meals that day, plus snacks, drinks and maybe afternoon tea; when your holiday clothes are feeling tight and you know you don't look as good as you'd like to in your bathing costume, then maybe you should forego the midnight buffet just this once. Or use the amazing facilities on board the ship – the gym, pool, sauna, spa, tennis court, games room and running circuit – to at least try to counterbalance some of the excesses. Instead, Aly and I found ourselves alone in the gym time and again. We were occasionally joined by other like-minded folk, none of whom needed to be there by the looks of them.

Years ago I would have found the idea of a daily workout quite a drag and would probably have given up after a few months, like a lot of people. Now, by running on a mental programme that tells me I love exercise and the rewards it brings, I really look forward to it and miss it terribly if something prevents me from doing it. Like the many clients I have helped over the years, you too can re-programme your mind in the same way so that when you are in a situation like we were on that cruise ship, you can truly enjoy the wonderful food and drink on offer but at the same time relish all the incredible opportunities at your disposal to improve your health as well, so that you return home relaxed, tanned, feeling supple and fit and so much better all round for the experience – as opposed to just being all round.

By using the exercise motivation technique below, which will help you develop a lasting motivation to get fit, you will never again think of exercise as a struggle. Instead, it will become second nature.

Learn how to enjoy exercise

Go to a quiet room where there are no distractions. Take a moment to get into a comfortable position, close your eyes and focus your attention on your breathing. Begin to breathe very slowly and deeply – in through your nose and out through your mouth. Make each breath long and deep, and feel your ribcage expand as you breathe in. Continue this for a short while until all the tension disappears from your body, and you feel relaxed.

Continue to breathe slowly and deeply in a steady, rhythmical, breathing pattern and when you reach the top of your breath hold it for three seconds, counting them out in your mind. Silently and mentally count to five on every out-breath. Relax more and more with every slow out-breath.

Now I want you to practise a more instant way of going into trance. Slowly and steadily count from one to three either silently or out loud. When you reach the number three say to yourself, 'I will become ten times more deeply relaxed.' You will go ten times deeper inside that powerful part of yourself where your true potential lies – your creativity, your courage and your self-belief. At the point you reach the number three go into a deeply relaxed state. Be more deeply relaxed than you've been in a long time. Every cell in your mind, body and spirit resonates with positive energy now. Take a short while to connect with this still, centred feeling.

Once you have finished the countdown, begin to create your visualization. Imagine yourself participating in exercise and feel yourself really enjoying it. It is important to use your emotions here so that you anchor a strong sense of enjoyment into your unconscious mind. Maybe visualize yourself on a treadmill or rowing machine, practising yoga, playing tennis, cycling, jogging or whatever works for you. As you see yourself doing this activity, connect with a feeling of pleasure and enjoyment. Make the visualization clear and use your senses to create a realistic mental image. Take a little time and let your imagination go.

After you have fully entered your visualization, I want you to repeat the following affirmations to yourself ten times or more in a slow, rhythmical way, almost like a chant. Say them with real feeling. Draw the phrases deep inside as you say them:

I love to exercise and keep fit.
**I go beyond old limitations and draw out my true
    potential.**
I deserve to be fit and healthy.
I live my life with courage and self-belief.

These affirmations are examples. Feel free to adapt them for your specific goals. You can even use the affirmations as a soundtrack to your visualization once you get the hang of it. Once you have stated and focused on your affirmations, you can compound these new beliefs by the counting method. Once again, count from one to three. This time, when you reach the number three, affirm that these positive new beliefs will sink ten times deeper into your unconscious mind and that the positive feelings will grow ten times stronger, ten times deeper inside into that powerful part of your self where your true potential lies. While slowly counting to three, feel yourself drawing your new beliefs deeply into your inner consciousness. Every cell in your mind, body and spirit is resonating with positive energy now. Take a moment to enjoy this feeling and to accept every new belief as a reality.

When you are ready, slowly count from one to ten, open your eyes and come back to full waking consciousness.

The more you move your body each day, the more energy you will have. The combination of healthy diet and regular exercise will make you feel so good that you won't want to go back to your old sluggish ways. This feel-good factor is quite addictive, as my television agent, Rob, will attest. Rob already enjoyed a good level of fitness and he came to me for help with his plans to run in the London Marathon. He had competed in a couple of marathons before, but wanted to go further and do better this time. With my help, harnessing his own willpower under hypnosis to make him push himself that little bit further, he was able not only to complete his remarkable challenge, but knock twenty minutes off his previous time, giving him a personal best of three hours, thirty minutes.

Now, you don't have to run a marathon, but you can start small and build yourself up to something that becomes a personal goal for you. It might be to win a game of tennis against an old adversary, or to row so many miles or run so many kilometres on the machines in the gym. You might hope to climb the ten flights of stairs to your office within a set time, or play a game of football with your son without running out of puff. Thinking of exercise in this challenging way is not only satisfying, it is incredibly self-motivating. You are taking back control of your life. You. Not me, or anyone else. You are improving your fitness, so that your chances of living to a ripe old age, and in good health, improve dramatically. So teach yourself well and see what a wonderful specimen of human determination you can be.

Golden rule 2
exercise and fitness

- Exercise each and every day of your life. Little and often is the key, even if it is simply walking or stretching. Mini-trampolines can provide a fantastic workout that takes little time and are great for increasing your metabolism.

- A ten-minute bounce first thing each morning will work wonders and you will be amazed at how your fitness will increase in a short space of time.

- Build regular exercise into your daily routines and work on developing a mindset that loves exercising. Get into a habit at least three times a week of indulging yourself in specific workouts at the gym, practising yoga, playing tennis, cycling, jogging or whatever appeals to you.

- Regular exercise will help you in so many ways and you absolutely must get into the habit of moving your body and being active on a daily basis.

Step 3

Positive mental attitude

'He who is of calm and happy nature will hardly feel the pressure of age, but to him who is of an opposite disposition youth and age are equally a burden.'

Plato

Boosting your self-esteem

Having a positive attitude has to be one of the best ways of keeping young, both physically and mentally. We all know the expression 'young at heart'. Someone who is happy and upbeat, physically active and able to make a valuable contribution to society is the antithesis of an older, unhealthy individual who sits at home, watching television, eating unhealthily and feeling miserable, while ageing visibly.

Negative thoughts are a part of what makes us

human. It is only natural to feel sad or unhappy about certain events that happen in our lives and to use those emotions to vent our feelings. The secret to feeling positive and happy, however, is not to dwell on them. There is a wonderful expression which is, 'Look back, but don't stare.' In other words, it's okay to remember bad things that have happened and to learn from them, but stop yourself constantly referring back to them or using them as the point of reference for the rest of your life. From now on you must view any mistakes, errors or unhappy experiences as lessons that will teach you something. Look for this lesson without wallowing or punishing yourself. The key is to learn the lesson so you don't make the same mistake again and to retain your self-belief by maintaining a positive internal dialogue.

In most cases, our feelings of positivity and self-worth are formed through our experiences in childhood. If you were never encouraged to love and respect yourself as a child, then you'll probably suffer low self-esteem in later life. This then leads you into all sorts of trouble, and ultimately allows others to walk all over you. An ancient Chinese lore claims that people are either warriors or victims. Warriors fight for what they want, remain focused and driven and often enjoy the power and control they've developed. Victims, on the other hand, go through life saying, 'Woe is me', and may even end up enjoying being downtrodden or victimized because it makes others feel sorry for them and treat them more kindly. It also absolves them from all responsibility. Much of what shapes either personality is the degree to which you love and respect yourself.

The first rule of learning to love and respect yourself is to banish any negativity from your mental vocabulary and stop it from getting in your way. Whenever a negative thought enters your brain let it drift away and focus instead on the positive. Think of your glass always as half-full, not half-empty. Self-criticism and doubt are extremely destructive, especially as your unconscious mind begins to accept the things you tell it. If you are forever berating yourself for being stupid or foolish, all you are doing is programming yourself to feel bad. You will then unconsciously respond to that negative programming and actually create situations for yourself that make you feel stupid or foolish. Remember, whatever you repeatedly affirm will become self-fulfilling.

By re-programming your personal 'computer' with positive beliefs about yourself, focusing on your successes rather than your failures, you will build more confidence and self-esteem. For example, you may not have reached the dizzy heights of the career path you once dreamed of, but you might be a wonderful mother, father, wife, husband, son, daughter, sister or brother. Being a good parent to your children is a huge success in life and highly underrated. Being kind, loving, compassionate and generous to friends and family are also desirable traits that everyone admires. If you have ever won or achieved anything, however small, don't be afraid to praise yourself. Maybe you are doing well at work, or you have reached some other personal goal. Always look at what you have achieved, acknowledge it, and be proud of yourself. There is nothing wrong with that; it is something you should embrace. You should also make a conscious effort to praise others, something which will not only make them feel better, but you too.

Banishing negativity

'Always aim at complete harmony of thought and word and deed ... aim at purifying your thoughts and everything will be well.'

Mahatma Gandhi

There are two hemispheres of the brain, which pass messages electronically between them. The right hemisphere, which is visual and processes information in an intuitive way, is believed to be responsible for imagination and creative thinking. The left brain processes that information logically and analytically and allows the human to respond in a rational way. Most people are dominated by one hemisphere or the other and tend, as they get older, to use the left brain more than the creative right brain, which is more active in childhood. Some people grow up to become what is known as 'whole-brained' and use both sides equally. It is widely accepted that the right brain holds the key to connecting with our inner talents and creativity, and that its use should be encouraged, especially when we are young and more closely in tune with its many functions. Once you begin to regularly express your creativity you will feel happier and less stressed, so it is important to cultivate the use of your creative brain functions. You can do this when you use self-hypnosis and visualization.

Many of us believe that the best way to relax is to get in from work and flop in front of the television, but finding a balance between watching TV and being creative is vital. Modern-day television programmes show a lot of negative images, especially in documentaries and news stories, not to mention soap operas that often focus on others' misfortunes. Newspapers are also full of negative stories – about war and death and natural disaster, the state of the country, the rising cost of living or the lottery of the health service. Be aware of how the media can be a negative influence on you, and not just with the content of their programmes or articles but with their advertising too.

Advertisers know how to manipulate and often incorporate mood music and persuasive language, especially when they want to promote unhealthy products or ideas. It seems every other ad is either for junk food or one featuring a compassionate-looking actor selling products or drugs for illnesses or ailments that more often than not have been caused by poor eating and lack of exercise in the first place. They are aimed at the very people who are watching – those sitting on their bums, eating rubbish and being taken in by the adverts, instead of switching the television off and going out to engage in something active or healthy. Magazines, too, play their part, especially those featuring countless images of celebrities of all ages looking amazing. The reality is that these pictures have often been doctored or airbrushed to make the subjects look slimmer, younger and generally more attractive. Or these wealthy individuals have repeatedly gone under the plastic surgeon's knife. Don't buy into this. You must never allow yourself to feel inadequate by measuring yourself against fake images. They are an illusion. Once you begin to look after yourself through healthy eating and exercise you will be able to avoid much of this hype and manipulation.

All this negativity and the urge to compare only creates fear and insecurity, which causes unhappiness. If you enjoy watching television, that's fine, but be selective about the programmes you choose. Don't buy magazines that feature only unrealistic or unattainable lifestyles.

Feeling more creative

Go to a quiet room where there are no distractions. Take a moment to get into a comfortable position, close your eyes and focus your attention on your breathing. Then begin breathing slowly and deeply – in through your nose and out through your mouth – in a circular motion. Breathe away any tension left in your body with every slow out-breath, and allow yourself to relax more and more.

Continue this breathing pattern a dozen or more times and clear away any unwanted thoughts until your mind becomes still and quiet. Don't worry if you get the odd unwanted thought; just re-centre your mind and allow the thought to drift away. Focus on the stillness of the moment. To guide yourself deeper into trance, silently and mentally count down from ten to one. Leave about five seconds between each number and feel every muscle in your body relax. Maybe you can imagine yourself going down a beautiful staircase or in an elevator with each descending number. Feel yourself drifting down into deeper and deeper levels of mental and physical relaxation when you get to this point; almost as though you are weightless, floating down through a dreamlike inner world – the inner world that leads to the genius inside you – the creative part of you.

Now as you lie there in this stillness, feeling centred and very calm, connect with a part of you that is responsible for your creativity: the childlike fun and creative part of you that is imaginative and carefree, that likes music and laughter. Take a moment to really feel this part of you and make a strong connection with it. Now silently ask this creative part of you for guidance. Take a couple of minutes to do this. Ask for ideas for new ventures. Don't force it – just allow the ideas to come. Sometimes you will get ideas and inspiration later. The key is that you connect with this creative part now and open up that channel. When you do this you will find inspiration within you and feel motivated to create and manifest new things in your life.

Allow five minutes to be still and centred and to allow your creative ideas to come forward. Affirm to yourself that you will feel more creative and inspired and that you can achieve many great things. State these affirmations as a reality now in the present tense:

- **I express my creativity in many different ways.**
- **I achieve many great things in my life.**
- **I draw opportunities towards me.**
- **I live life with great courage.**
- **I believe in myself and in my own ability.**

As you state these phrases, draw the words inside you and really believe them. You may want to add your own. When you are ready, allow your mind to clear and count slowly upwards from one to ten, and open your eyes and come back to full waking consciousness: ... 1 ... 2 ... 3 ... 4 ... 5 ... 6 ... 7 ... 8 ... 9 ...10 ... Practise this exercise often, especially when you are looking for ideas or inspiration.

Take up some creative right-brain pursuits instead, like gardening or sports, art, DIY or crafts. Join a pub quiz or read a book. If you have children, make a conscious effort to limit their TV viewing or magazine-flicking too and get them into the habit of doing something more creative, preferably with you. If you ingrain these principles into children from an early age it can have a profound knock-on effect, and they will grow up to become brighter, more creative adults.

Positive modelling

'Don't bother just to be better than your contemporaries or predecessors. Try to be better than yourself.'

William Faulkner

As human beings we often seek to validate our behaviour weaknesses and bad habits. We sometimes do this by choosing friends who have similar unhealthy habits, because it allows us to feel okay about our own behaviour. If you are twenty-five pounds overweight and you have a friend who is forty pounds overweight then it can be easy to justify your excesses by saying, 'I'm not as bad as so-and-so.' Similarly, if we are unhappy and negative but know someone who is even more so, we can always reassure ourselves that we have not sunk to their depths yet.

I'm not saying you should dump all your overweight, unhappy or unhealthy friends, but don't judge yourself against others who are weak-willed and content to stay stuck in a rut. Worse than that, they may even hold you back, keen to have someone like them around to make them feel better. You must aspire to modelling yourself on people who are happy, fit and healthy, if that is what you really want.

The following metaphor sums up what I am saying: a man goes into a restaurant where he notices a large bucket of live crabs. One crab is climbing up the bucket wall and looks like it is going to escape, so the man informs the waiter. The waiter tells the man that the crab will never escape, as every time it gets near to the top the other crabs in the bucket always pull it back. The moral to this story is never to allow others to hold you back. You are going to achieve your target goals and become happier and more fulfilled, regardless of what anyone else says or thinks or does. Even though you may encounter some resistance and negativity on your journey, you will also secretly inspire people and many will be very proud of you.

The following is a technique that will help you learn to assimilate the same qualities held by someone who inspires you. To start with, you must imagine a friend, relative or acquaintance who is a positive, happy person, who eats healthily, exercises regularly and has a lifestyle and appearance you aspire to. Choose someone you know and see fairly often. Set your goal high. If you can't think of any friends who fit the bill, imagine a famous person you admire who does.

Gratitude is always a good place to start when you want to feel more positive. It is all too easy to pay attention to what is wrong in our lives or to the things that don't work. Focus now on all the things that do work for you. If you are fortunate enough to be healthy in your mind, body and spirit, for example, take a moment to give thanks for that. If you have perfect use of your arms and legs and the ability to walk, run, read, write, hear, see and talk, then you are lucky. Many people don't have these simple blessings and to have the ability to do one or more of these things would be their ultimate wish.

If ever you get stuck in a negative rut or feel down about something, read the book or listen to the recordings by Christopher Reeve, the *Superman* actor who was critically injured in a horse-riding accident. After his fall, he was paralysed from the neck down and needed a machine just to help him breathe. He fought against his disability until the day he died, writing books and producing recordings documenting his epic struggle. When you read or hear what being quadriplegic is like,

Modelling technique

Allow yourself to become comfortable and close your eyes. Breathe slowly and deeply, in through your nose and out through your mouth. Make each breath long and deep, and relax more and more with every slow out-breath. Focus on your role model. Take a moment to see this person in your mind's eye, and focus on their levels of happiness, health and fitness. Concentrate on the qualities you like about them. Take a moment to feel inspired.

Now imagine that all of these qualities are becoming part of you. Feel as though you are drawing their positive mental attitude, determination and discipline deep inside yourself. Embrace their good habits as your own. Make these a part of you now. Visualize yourself achieving your happiness and fitness goal with the same self-belief and determination as the person you admire. You are in control of your life now and determined to become and remain fit, toned and healthy in the same way they have, prolonging your life and improving your appearance. Take a moment to focus on this. Be creative and use all of your senses when you visualize yourself

> expressing the new characteristics that will help you to achieve and maintain a high level of contentment.
>
> Take all the time you need to do this. When you are ready to finish, allow your mind to clear and slowly count from one to three. Open your eyes and come back to full waking consciousness.

you will feel completely differently about your ability to get up out of your chair and walk across the room. You will see it as a huge gift. Whenever you feel stuck in a rut, do something charitable or seek out inspirational books, recordings, films, all of which will help you to reframe your perspective.

Think, too, of that great movie *It's a Wonderful Life* starring James Stewart. A man whose life seems to have gone awry through no fault of his own throws himself off a bridge and is rescued from drowning by an angel. The angel grants him his wish that he is dead. When he comes to, the man returns home to find nothing as it was. His wife is an unhappy spinster. His lovely children have never been born. His influence on friends and family, even on how his town took shape, has all been lost. He is confronted with a grim and unfriendly world, which quickly makes him realize that – no matter how imperfect his life seemed – he was one of the most fortunate people he knew and made a real contribution to others. Desperate to find the angel again, he is finally granted a second wish that he is no longer dead and returns home with an entirely new and positive outlook, embracing and celebrating all that he has, instead of being miserable about what he thought he didn't have.

Never take your health, happiness and well-being for granted. Make a point on waking each morning of focusing on all the blessings in your life, whatever they may be, such as your family, your health, your relationships and friendships, your house and your job. Later on you can focus on achieving more and setting goals, but wherever you are in your life, having a good dose of gratitude will help you feel more positive.

We each have so much talent and brilliance inside us; every single one of us has unique abilities and infinite creativity that we should regularly embrace and praise ourselves for. The key is in learning how to connect with our unique inner potential and to draw it out. The techniques, ideas and teachings in this book will help you to do just that. Hypnotherapy can be extremely effective in releasing negative conditioning. The following story is a good example of what can be achieved:

Positive mental attitude
case study

A client came to see me who was an alcoholic desperate to be free of his drink problem. He was stuck in a destructive and negative pattern of behaviour that had been going on for eight years. He was drinking a bottle of vodka a day and had become aggressive and abusive to those close to him. Paradoxically, although he was a tough guy, he was also very emotional. During an in-depth consultation, he made a vague connection between the onset of his problems and a car crash eight years previously in which someone in another car had died.

I guided him into a relaxed state and regressed him back to the accident. He was in no way to blame but was nevertheless tormented with guilt. When I regressed him further it transpired that on the evening of the accident he had promised his son that he would be at his school speech day to see him collect an award. Instead, he worked late and didn't make it. On his way home, he was involved in the accident. In his deepest thoughts, he focused on the negatives and saw the accident as his punishment. In the trance state he told me, 'If I hadn't stayed late, it wouldn't have happened.' His feelings were complicated and compounded by the suppressed guilt he felt at letting his son down.

Unable to face his demons, he had tried to blot out his memories of that night with drink. Having hypnotized him, I guided him to resolve this inner conflict and release his guilt. At the end of the session he wept and felt massive relief. He couldn't wait to get home to his family and, as he put it, 'start to make up for being such an arsehole'. With just one regression he was able to resolve his inner conflict and free himself of his self-destructive behaviour.

When I saw him a month or so later he looked totally different. He had not touched any alcohol and had no desire to go back to it. He lost two stone in weight and looked happy, healthy and full of life. He told me his wife wanted to thank me for giving her her husband back.

This is a dramatic story but it demonstrates how people get stuck in negative patterns that hold them back or, worse, destroy them. It also shows how easy it can often be to overcome such problems. When we store memories, we store the associated emotions as well. If you go through a trauma and it becomes repressed, the memory and the connected emotions sometimes get stuck. If something triggers that memory years later, the emotions that accompany it are also released. This can be very confusing if you don't understand what is happening or why.

The effect of music is a positive example of this. When you hear a song that reminds you of a time when you fell in love years before, just hearing it again can bring back the same romantic feelings. Couples often look adoringly at each other and say, 'This is our song', when a particular record comes on. Or when the soundtrack for an especially memorable movie is played, you feel a stirring in your heart and are taken right back to the high emotion of the moment. For some people, music can have the opposite effect. Because of my rough childhood, I often joke that when I hear an old song by The Sex Pistols or The Clash, I want to start a fight or smash up a telephone box. It is a light-hearted way of saying the same thing – memories and emotions are intertwined in such a way that is often confusing and complicated. With hypnotherapy or self-improvement techniques, however, these emotions can be harnessed to produce good feelings, viewed from the perspective of distance that can ultimately have an enormously positive influence on your life.

Happy hormones

'All the days of the oppressed are wretched
but the cheerful heart has a continual feast.'

Proverbs 15:15

Scientists and doctors have discovered that our emotional health is inexorably linked to our physical well-being and ability to heal ourselves. Cancer patients shown funny movies over a prolonged period of time have been known to release so many endorphins and positive chemicals into their bodies that they have cured themselves – quite literally – by laughing themselves better. Researchers have even found that you can achieve the same positive biological and physiological effects by forcing a smile, rather than wearing one naturally. Never mind about 'smile lines'; smiling and laughing boost the immune system and do you the power of good.

Inspired by this research, laughter clubs have sprung up all over the world, where people gather and encourage themselves and each other to laugh out loud at jokes and stories. They do exercises that open the chest and increase lung capacity; they sing and dance and do anything they can think of to promote a positive mental attitude. There are now thousands of laughter therapy programmes in hospitals, old people's homes and prisons to fight depression and stress, and laughtercising classes for those wanting to tighten tummy muscles and keep fit. Therapists call it 'internal jogging'. You can buy recordings of other people laughing uproariously just to make you laugh along with them, so beneficial are the biological results. There are weight-loss books that claim that by laughing out loud for at least thirty seconds up to ten times a day you will be guaranteed to lose food cravings, develop more energy and become so positive that exercise and other creative activities seem more appealing.

Immersing yourself in the positive experience of cheerfulness can undoubtedly help your body look and feel younger. If you work too hard, feel unfit, or take your life so seriously that there is no room for joy to fill your heart and enrich your daily existence, then you might as well be old and decrepit because – sooner rather than later – that's exactly what you will be. Make a commitment to be positive and bring joy to yourself and others, and it will happen.

'Smile and the world smiles with you', the song goes. 'Cry and you cry alone.' Never a truer word was spoken.

Golden rule 3
positive mental
attitude

- When you create a strong positive mental outlook you will be able to deal with stress and the pressures of life. Having goals to aim for is crucial for creating a positive outlook. If you don't have ambitions then life happens to you rather than you creating the life you want.

- To create a positive future you have to believe your future is golden in the first place. Even if things are not how you want them to be now, you can always change them. You do this not through wishing or yearning, which is weak and ineffective, but through positive visualization and creating strong inner beliefs that your future will be everything you want it to be.

- Write down a list of goals for your personal life and one for your work or career. List ten clear goals for each, in the present tense, as though they are a reality now. When making your lists, make sure you set a time frame for all the goals to be achieved. Print them out and place them wherever you can see them.

- Surround yourself with positive people who have similar ambitions and who inspire you and avoid people who drain your energy.

Step 4

Healthy sleeping patterns

'Sleep that knits up the ravelled sleeve of care
The death of each day's life, sore labour's bath
Balm of hurt minds, great nature's second course
Chief nourisher in life's feast.'

William Shakespeare

Beauty sleep

People who sleep well live longer, and that is a well-documented medical fact. We all know how great we feel after a good night's sleep, and how much better we look. Sleeping at least six to eight hours a night every night helps your body to heal itself, builds up the immune system, lowers blood pressure and reduces the risk of weight gain and diabetes.

According to Francesco Cappuccio, Professor of

Epidemiology and Cardiovascular Medicine at Warwick Medical School in the UK, 'There is a clear connection between sleep and health, sleep deprivation and disease – and the evidence is getting stronger.' A study of ten thousand people at Warwick discovered that reducing sleep to five hours or fewer on a regular basis doubles the risk of dying from cardiovascular disease. Other studies have found that the sleep-deprived produce more stress hormones – which have been linked to everything from migraines and stomach problems to cancer – and fewer growth hormones, which give you better skin and muscle mass.

When sleep problems occur over a long period of time they can rapidly speed up the ageing process. The parallels between sleeplessness and ageing are in part because the effects of both impair the pre-frontal cortex – the region of your brain that is most active when you are awake. Lack of sleep has also been shown to cause skin disorders in both animals and humans. Another less obvious problem aggravated by sleep deprivation is the onset of 'man-boobs' and pot bellies in middle-aged men. The reason is that men produce their growth hormone almost exclusively when they sleep. When a man is sleep-deprived, his body will not be producing enough of the growth hormone as required. Scientists believe that falling growth hormone production is a factor in turning muscles into flab. So for men to avoid blobbing out in middle age good sleep is a must, which highlights yet another reason why the quality of your sleep is so important.

Long ago our ancestors would rise when it was light and work, rest and play during daylight hours, then wind down as the night approached and sleep when it became dark. They followed the natural rhythms of the day and night and probably slept soundly because of it. The statistics in this round-the-clock world of ours where the importance of sleep has been slowly eroded are frightening. More than one in four people suffers from problems sleeping on a regular basis and many go on to develop chronic insomnia, which often leads to depression and poor performance at work and home. An estimated three thousand serious injuries or deaths are caused by road accidents brought about by fatigue (although that figure could be much higher), as loss of sleep affects everything from decision-making and mood to productivity and moral judgement. People who get insufficient sleep double their risk of obesity, not only because of growth hormones but because they are awake longer and later at a time when food cravings and the need for sugar to raise insulin levels often kick in.

On average, we spend a third of our lives asleep and use that time to re-energize and rejuvenate. The brain and body enter into an inactive restful state and allow information that has been amassed during the day to be absorbed and digested. Sleep has a major impact on brain development and affects everything from memory to speech. These facilities quickly become impaired without regular, healthy sleep.

Quite apart from our inability to think straight as well as feeling lethargic and irritable, we have all looked in the mirror after a bad night's sleep and seen the dark rings under our eyes, or the way our skin looks sallow and grey. Just one disturbed night ages us visibly. Being overloaded with mental pressures often makes it difficult to switch off once we go to bed and in our technologically advanced world with twenty-four-hour television and shops and bars open all hours there are plenty of excuses to fight against the natural rhythms of our body. Yet even though we know and understand how damaging sleep deprivation can be, many people still don't address the underlying causes and carry on inflicting mental torture on themselves while under-mining their physical health.

I know, because I did just that for a number of years. Despite having turned my life around in terms of healthy eating and lifestyle, sleep was the last nut I had to crack and a problem I only resolved relatively recently. After years of being in the music business, never getting to bed until the early hours, I acquired bad sleep habits and continued to live like a vampire long after I left the industry. Going to bed when the rest of the house was asleep became the norm for me, as did lying in late – particularly if I'd had a restless night. After years of treating others with sleep problems, the penny finally dropped and I began to realize how damaging this was for me, health-wise and emotionally. I made a conscious effort to alter my customary bedtime rituals and go to bed at a reasonable hour like everyone else. It took a few weeks to get into a new rhythm but I now make sleep a top priority that nothing gets in the way of. I follow the rule that an hour before midnight is worth two after. As a result, I feel fitter, healthier and have far more energy, especially in the mornings when I now do most of my fitness workouts.

Hypnosis and sleep

'A ruffled mind makes a restless pillow.'

Charlotte Brontë

Hypnosis is the perfect tool for relaxing the body and quietening the mind. By slowing your brainwaves to the levels they would reach in sleep, you are allowing your brain to switch off and shut down more quickly than it would do naturally if you are anxious or have too many things on your mind. It is far better than turning to drugs, which can become addictive and have long term side-effects that can undo the benefits they might temporarily bring.

During an eight-hour sleep cycle, we switch between two different sleep states – REM or rapid eye movement sleep for the lesser part of any sleeping time, and non-REM sleep for the longer periods, when we are more deeply asleep. REM sleep is akin to the state you are in when you are under hypnosis. The eyeballs start to move around beneath the eyelids, which is always a good indicator to the therapist that the subject is in a deep hypnotic trance. Dreams mostly happen during REM sleep and throughout the night we go through a repeated cycle of the two different sleep types.

Most people need between six and eight hours' sleep a night or we begin to accumulate what is known as 'sleep debt', which builds like a financial debt and cannot be paid off without extra sleep in the form of a lie-in or a restful holiday. Recent studies have shown that in order to 'pay back' this debt, you have to sleep for half the amount of time owed, although it varies from person to person. Some people never quite catch up, become overtired during the day and find themselves cat-napping, or even falling asleep when they shouldn't. Sleep deprivation directly affects co-ordination and concentration, and this mental fatigue can be extremely dangerous if we are driving or doing something that

The beauty sleep supercharge

- Do not drink any coffee, tea or alcohol and avoid anything laden with sugar or salt.
- Drink lots of water during the day but avoid drinking too much late at night so that you don't wake needing the lavatory.
- Exercise as much as possible, winding down with something gentle like yoga or Pilates at the end of the day and at least three hours before your bedtime.
- During the day, avoid indigestible items or anything that will stimulate your body or cause your stomach to churn all night.
- Cut down your television viewing or computer use in the evening.
- Have a warm bath before you go to bed. Add a sprinkle of fresh lavender or lavender oil to your pillow.
- Go to bed early – preferably before eleven o'clock at night.
- Once your head is on the pillow, visualize the following day's events in a positive light. See yourself looking and feeling great. See the future event visualization technique on page 15.
- Breathe deeply, in through your nose and out through your mouth, allowing your body to relax from the top of your head to the tip of your toes. Feel yourself sinking deeply into the mattress and your pillow. Relax.

requires us to be fully present. Used as a form of torture in certain countries, sleep deprivation weakens the mind's ability to resist interrogation and makes prisoners far more vulnerable.

Sadly, having too much sleep doesn't make us any younger, however – in fact, people who sleep more than ten hours each night have a higher than average risk of dying prematurely, so it is important to get the balance right. To make sure you have a good night's sleep before an important day, follow these steps to ensure that your night is as restful as it can be.

Sleep disorders are some of the most common problems I deal with, as hypnotherapy is such an effective tool for guiding people into healthy sleeping patterns. Once hypnosis has led you into a state of altered consciousness akin to sleep, a suggestion like 'As soon as your head hits the pillow, you will fall into a deep and relaxing sleep, waking refreshed and alert in the morning' will be accepted into your unconscious mind that much more easily. When your head next hits the pillow, the suggestion becomes your reality. Using the audio and your own techniques you can learn to create the natural states of pre- and post-sleep at will and induce your own suggestions quite easily.

Insomnia, which is the Latin word for sleeplessness, is estimated to affect around twenty per cent of the population annually, mostly women. Causes can be anything from depression, anxiety, stress, fear and pain to an overactive imagination. External factors include caffeine, noise or light disturbance, an uncomfortable bed, eating too much too late, constipation, fluctuations in temperature or going to bed hungry. For many of us, transient insomnia is something, as its name suggests, that occurs every now and again. It usually lasts from a single night to a few weeks. Acute insomnia is the next stage up and can last up to several weeks, while chronic insomnia occurs every night for at least a month and seriously impairs physical and mental health. Sufferers usually end up relying on medication.

Whichever type people suffer from, insomnia is a symptom of a problem and not a disease. In almost every case, a lifestyle change or some gentle hypnotherapy as part of a natural, holistic approach can correct the problem. The root causes of some of these sleeping problems are often unique to a person's past experience so the solutions are different in every case. The key is to learn to relax, which is helped by a healthy diet and the possession of a fit, exercised body, plus developing a positive mental attitude and an uncluttered, stress-free mind. Most of all, you must learn to revere your sleep and never underestimate its importance. Make sure that this becomes a priority in your life and organize yourself around facilitating a good sleep every night.

The following technique is ideal if you are feeling

Self-hypnosis recharge

If you are not getting enough sleep and don't have the opportunity to catch up on your sleep debt use self-hypnosis during the day. A lunchtime break at work is an ideal opportunity, so directly after you have eaten go to a quiet place and get into a comfortable position, preferably lying down. Don't worry if there are distractions nearby; just calm your mind by closing your eyes and breathing slowly and deeply in through your nose and out through your mouth.

Feel all the muscles in your body relax with each slow out-breath and allow your mind to become still and quiet. Stay in this still space for at least fifteen minutes or as long as feasible. You can use this or any of the longer self-hypnosis techniques in this book if you have more time. After ten or twenty minutes of being in this calm and centred space you will feel energized, clearer in your mind, and much more effective in your work. You will also go some way towards clearing your sleep debt.

tired during the day at your office or workplace and you need to recharge.

Former Prime Minister Margaret Thatcher got by on an average of four hours' sleep a night, but made up her

Sleep case study 1

Sleep problems can stem from a wide variety of causes and one of my most unusual sessions was with a lady who came to see me because she had a fear of the dark which was keeping her awake. She explained that as soon as night fell, she would become anxious and sometimes have panic attacks. She had tried other therapies and medical help without success.

I followed a technique to regress the lady back to cause of her problem. When she was in a deeply relaxed state I told her, 'When I count to three, you will go back to the first time you experienced fear of the dark.' To my surprise she regressed back to a past life in ancient Egypt in which she was in a dark temple. She told me that there were all kinds of rituals going on, including sacrifices to appease the gods. The story she relayed was vivid and detailed. Then an amazing thing happened, which I have never seen before or since. She began speaking in a foreign language. I don't speak Egyptian but it seemed to me to be Arabic or some similar language from that part of the world.

I was amazed but remained focused and was able to guide her to let go of any negative emotions connected to

this experience. I also reinforced the suggestions that she
would now be free of the fear of the dark. At the right time
I guided her back to full consciousness. On waking, she
confirmed that she did not speak any other language and
had little recollection of being in a trance. She also felt she
had only been under for five minutes when she had in fact
been in a trance for an hour.

When she returned for a second session a week later
she told me that for the first time in years she was now able
to sleep through the night without any fear. Whether or not
she had really experienced a past life or just had a vivid
imagination was not for me to judge. What was important
to me was that the fear had gone and her problem had
been solved.

sleep debt by doing something similar to the above
technique for twenty minutes each day and ensuring she
had at least one good night's sleep a week. Love her or
loathe her, she got a lot done on just four hours' sleep a
night.

And so to bed

'Silence is the sleep that nourishes wisdom.'

Francis Bacon

Many people do not revere their sleep nearly as much as they should. Nor do they make their bedrooms the comfortable sanctuaries of tranquillity and calm that they should be. Children and pets should most definitely be banned and you should pay special attention to making the environment in which you will, after all, be spending a third of your life as soothing as possible.

Decorate your bedroom in soft colours conducive to relaxation and sleep, such as green, blue or lilac. Colours that have a stimulating effect like bright reds, oranges or yellows should be avoided. Make sure there is soft lighting and, ideally, buy a natural daylight alarm clock where the light slowly turns off at night to mimic the sunset and in the morning gives off a similar effect to sunrise. Ensure that your bedroom is as quiet and dark as possible. Thick curtains are a good idea if you live in an area with a lot of noise. To eliminate all noise and light consider using ear-plugs, black-out blinds and a sleep mask. These can also help if your partner snores or comes to bed at a later time than you.

Your bed must be comfortable and your mattress,

pillows and sheets clean. Turn your mattress every six months and wash your sheets regularly. Invest in some really good quality bed linens and pillows. Make sure you are not too warm or too cold. Don't have too many covers or a duvet that is too heavy but also make sure your covers don't leave you feeling chilly. If you live in an environment that is polluted, buy a natural air-purifying device for your bedroom. Avoid watching television in the evening for at least two nights a week, or as often as you can. Read a book instead or spend a relaxing evening doing things that won't stimulate your mind. Even if you can do this once or twice a week it is probable that you will sleep better on the nights when your brain is not bombarded with imagery. Try it and see how different it feels.

I suggested all these changes to a client with chronic insomnia who once came to me. He had tried many solutions in the past but nothing had helped. On gentle examination, he admitted that his bedroom was more like a home entertainment centre than a place of sanctuary – it had a wide-screen television, a hi-fi, a computer and all manner of gadgets that were undoubtedly polluting the air with electromagnetic transmissions and distracting him from the important business of sleeping. After clearing out all this equipment, improving his lifestyle habits through diet, exercise and the avoidance of stimulants, and having some personalized hypnotherapy to help him relax, he ended up sleeping six to eight hours every night instead of the two he had been averaging for years. His case was typical of so many people I help and goes to show that,

Calming your mind

Go to a quiet room where there are no distractions. Light a candle and place it in front of you. Switch off all the lights so that the candle flame provides the only light. Sit comfortably and focus on the flickering flame. Watch the way it dances in the air and begin to breathe slowly and deeply, in through your nose and out through your mouth in a circular motion until your mind becomes still and centred.

Keeping your eyes on the flame, be in the here and now and accept everything that is. With every slow intake of breath, allow yourself to relax further and focus your mind only on the flame. Banish unwanted thoughts as you watch the flame move and its colour change. Remain in this pleasant, relaxed state as long as you like. Do not underestimate the power of this simple technique, which clears the mind and focuses on only what is directly in front of you. When you are ready, blow out the candle and close your eyes. Remain seated, in the darkness, centred and relaxed and avoid all extraneous thought. After a minute or so, make your way to bed and sleep well and deeply.

using a holistic approach, the problems people often believe they are stuck with all their lives can be solved.

Avoid stress as much as possible by meditating, playing a gentle sport, or practising yoga, Pilates or Tai Chi especially in the evenings. Calm your mind to alleviate tension before you go to bed, either by listening to soothing music, doing some sort of relaxation exercise or by using the following technique which is fantastic at helping you wind down thirty minutes or so before you retire to bed.

Many people with sleep problems become dependent on sleeping pills, or use alcohol or other drugs to try to get their bodies to relax before they go to bed. There is no need for anything other than the key steps listed in this book to help anyone sleep, but for those who favour a more holistic approach and would like to try natural remedies in addition to the techniques learned here, there are a few I would recommend. Meditation and relaxation are useful, but aromatherapy, reflexology, homeopathy and acupuncture are also said to be beneficial. Self-administered herbal treatments such as chamomile, lavender, valerian, aniseed, hops, rauwolfia and passion flower can be taken in teas, last thing at night, or used as essential oils in a warm bath. A daily vitamin B supplement is said to improve relax-ation by adding thiamine to the nervous system, and pomegranates and lettuce are said to help insomniacs

Sleep case study 2

A woman came to me not long ago with a serious case of fatigue. Even though she fell asleep easily, she felt exhausted when she woke up and her husband reported that she was often restless in the night, calling out. Under hypnosis I was able to regress her back to the cause of her problem, which was a childhood experience of sexual abuse that had happened in the middle of the night and which she had largely blocked from her mind.

With her permission and my help, she revisited the experience, this time from the safety and comfort of adulthood, knowing that she survived the ordeal and that it never happened again. She had what is known as an 'abreaction' – a release of emotions or trauma stored in the memory – which was extremely cathartic for her. During our sessions, these unhappy memories and emotions were not only released but logically processed until she felt purged of the experience.

Within a few weeks she was sleeping normally for the first time in years and woke each morning feeling refreshed and renewed. Her husband thanked me in person – for the first time in their marriage he, too, was getting a good night's sleep.

sleep. Two teaspoons of organic honey in a large cup of hot water four hours before going to bed is said to have a hypnotic action and induce a sound sleep.

Worry is a big cause of sleep disorders as people lie awake, tossing and turning, fretting about everything from their financial status or the future of their children to the threat of impending world war. Using the calming the mind technique (see page 103) will be beneficial, as will the general changes to a healthy diet and lifestyle that will help you relax and feel ready for bed when the time comes. To worry at night is probably one of the worst things you can do, because it creates fear and blocks any positive energy at the time when it is most needed. That positive energy is what will help lift you from whatever situation it is that is causing your concern in the first place, so if you are blocking it, you are preventing yourself from reaping its benefits. Focus your energy instead on creating a world in which you feel happy and comfortable, and in which your ability to sleep long, well and deeply each night will recharge you and allow you to face the challenges of the days ahead.

If possible, always try to imagine the best case scenario, rather than the worst. See yourself healthy and happy, your life full of abundance and contentment. Allow yourself the joy of this vision and create pictures in your mind of how it will look and be. The more you feel and believe how the future could look the more likely it will be to happen. Banish negative thoughts as the demons that are trying to undermine your confidence and self-esteem. Use affirmations to confirm how many blessings you already have and to imagine how many more you will have in the future.

Cherish your sleep and come to understand its importance in creating a new, better life for you and those around you. Most of all, focus on all that you are doing now that is positive and healthy in changing your lifestyle and eradicating previously negative patterns to look younger and live longer.

Golden rule 4
sleep

- Get into the habit of going to bed at the same time every night, the earlier the better. Remember – an hour before midnight is worth two after.

- Remove any televisions, hi-fi equipment, mobile phones or landline telephones from your bedroom. Your bedroom is for sleeping and its environment should be conducive to sleep.

- Sleep in complete darkness so that not even the light from your alarm clock can be seen. Make sure you turn off any lights outside your room. Use black-out blinds if necessary, to block out the morning light.

- Do not eat or drink anything other than water or herbal tea for at least four hours before you go to bed.

- Keep a notepad and pen by your bedside so that you can jot down things you need to do the next day. Once you have written them on your pad you can forget about them and go to sleep safe in the knowledge that what you have written down will be remembered. Keeping such a list will help you switch off from any worries and go to sleep feeling more organized. If you tend to mull over problems or get unwanted thoughts at night then you must also use the calming your mind technique on page 103.

Step 5

Financial security and career contentment

'The future depends on what we do in the present.'

Mahatma Gandhi

Finding your way

Now that we have covered the four key steps to looking younger and living longer, we move on to the other factors that, although not quite so important, can also have an important effect on the way you look, feel and live your daily life. Some of them may relate to you and some may not. The first of these is financial security and career contentment.

We all know what we look and feel like when we are stressed. New, tight lines appear on our faces, lack of sleep through worry or a busy mind dulls our eyes and makes our skin sallow, and our whole bodies feel tense.

One of the chief causes of stress and anxiety is money. A close second is job satisfaction or, rather, lack of it. If we can eliminate these concerns or at least alleviate them, then the stress that ages us and makes us feel weighed down will lift, and we will be able to begin a new phase more hopeful and lighter in spirit.

My own story is probably the best I know as an example of how to create financial security and career contentment. I had a best mate from childhood called Terry; a lad who came from the same neighbourhood. During our teens we took different paths in life. My ego pulled me in the hedonistic direction of the pop world while his focus was on achieving financial success. Having been offered fame and fortune as a teenager through the music business, I then lost everything through bad decisions and my various addictions and spent the next ten years scratching a living. Terry and I lost touch for several years but met up again in our mid-twenties when we discovered we were living near each other in south London. In contrast to me, Terry had become a self-made millionaire and was on the Rich List of top earners. He lived in a luxury penthouse apartment in an up-market area, while three miles away I was living miserably at the top of a council tower block.

We met for a drink a couple of times but it was difficult to re-connect. I joked that we'd both rocketed with similar speed to opposite ends of the social scale.

Secretly, his meteoric rise made me feel a complete failure. I believed then, however, as I believe now, that you make your own success in life. Meeting up with Terry again made me refocus on my life and become more determined to succeed. Fear of failure was a great motivator. I pondered what it was that had taken our lives in such different directions when we had started as equals. After some self-analysis, I figured it out – Terry was disciplined and I was lazy; he was determined and I had been half-hearted. Where he had belief in himself, I had none.

That realization was a turning point for me. From that day on, I decided to change my attitude and raise my game. I didn't know how or where to begin but I did become extremely determined to make something of myself and fight the label of 'waster' I'd been stuck with since childhood. Through trial and error, I eventually pulled myself out of my slumber and forged ahead with my new goals. Whatever your motivation is, find it and use it to fire yourself up. Always remember: the only way you can fail is if you quit.

Remaining focused

'Be great in act, as you have been in thought.'

William Shakespeare

When I eventually got the fire in my belly, I started with the basics, by getting rid of everything that was holding me back. I began on a programme of improving my mind and body. I started to read more, especially self-help titles, to inspire and educate me. I also began associating with positive people and gently moved away from anyone who was a drain on my energy. It was a lonely road at times. When you start to make changes in yourself, even positive ones, you may find your relationships change. People around you can start to feel insecure or see their own shortcomings thrown into sharp relief. They may even fear losing the 'old' you. The key is to move on regardless, not in a ruthless way, just not allowing yourself to be pulled back because of others' insecurities. Those who really care about you will eventually come around if they see that what you are doing is for the right reasons. You will win their respect in the end.

When I first started as a hypnotherapist I set myself clear goals, writing them down. My chief aim was to sell one hundred thousand of my hypnosis tapes within three years. I remember looking at this and thinking 'Wouldn't that be great?' but a part of me didn't really believe it was possible as a self-published, one-man-band. I was recording the tapes on a set-up in the back bedroom of my tiny, two-bedroom terraced house. I then duplicated the cassettes one at a time and printed each cover on a home printer. I made display cabinets from wood I bought in B&Q and sold the tapes to local shops. I worked hard and within two years, I had reached my target. It felt really good to know that I was the master my own destiny through my own focused efforts. Using Terry as my inspiration, I had forced myself to change my lazy, unfocused ways and altered my life forever.

The momentum of that first clear statement of intent carried the project further than I could ever have imagined. When you create goals and reach them, your belief in what you can achieve in the future becomes stronger. At first it feels like you are turning the tide and things happen slowly, but as your energy grows, you can manifest things much more quickly and easily.

Coping with financial stress

'Annual income twenty pounds, annual expenditure nineteen six, result happiness. Annual income twenty pounds, annual expenditure twenty
pound ought and six, result misery.'

Charles Dickens

Worrying about money – whether you have enough or
even have too much – can be a major source of stress.
This in turn creates negativity that blocks you enjoying
what you have and will make you old before your time.
Most people believe that having a lot of money would
solve all their problems but I know millionaires who are
utterly miserable. How about those lottery winners who
claim that money destroyed their lives? It is not their
good fortune that messed them up, but their attitude
to it and their inability to cope with their change of
circumstances.

Whether you are rich or poor, you have to learn to
develop a relaxed and positive attitude towards money.
Even if you live in a crumbling tower block, as I once
did, don't buy into the 'poor me' syndrome. With a
little desire and determination you can always raise the
quality of your life. Don't fret about not having money,
as this will only block your natural abundance and create

Success case studies

A friend who is a singer/songwriter told me that when she learnt about self-hypnosis and the power of affirmations she would regularly affirm that she would have a number one hit. Every day she would get herself into a centred state and visualize this scenario in colourful detail. Within one year of starting this discipline in the mid-nineties, she wrote a song with her partner that went to number one in the British charts and now has a gold disk proudly displayed on her wall.

A customer from Scotland wrote to thank me after buying a book and audio recording I had compiled about creating wealth and abundance. In his letter, he said the results had been 'quite frankly amazing'. Since beginning listening to the audio and practising the techniques, he said great things have happened to him. 'I've moved from an awful flat into a really nice one. I have had debt wiped out. I was given a computer, and a year's broadband. I have begun a five-year plan to radically change my life. And now I have started work on songs for an album, two movie scripts and a comedy sitcom I am writing. Plus I volunteer on local community radio, for which we won an award. I am gaining broadcasting experience. All the dreams I thought I'd left

behind at seventeen are starting to come together again.
Plus my mates are nonplussed that I keep winning money
on the lottery! You are an inspiration, Glenn. God bless you,
bro.'

Anything you want is just waiting for you to step up and
claim it.

unnecessary suffering. Yearning for anything is a waste
of energy. Instead you have to be clear in your aims and
take action.

As this man and so many others have discovered, if
you are in debt or spending too much, you need to rid
yourself of this type of destructive behaviour. Look into
the reasons behind such patterns. Is your desire to
overspend driven by something in your past? Are you
trying to keep up with others? Are you depressed and
trying to make yourself feel better? Once you get to the
bottom of what drives you to overspend then you can
change that behaviour. If you are depressed, for example,
do something active and enjoyable that is free, like
taking a walk or going for a swim, rather than heading
for the shops. This is a holistic journey and these little
steps will help you to create a happier and less stressed
lifestyle.

How to get out of debt and release financial stress

Step 1. Write two lists, one detailing your total monthly income and the other listing all your monthly outgoings. Look at new ways to make sure your income exceeds your outgoings. Don't fret if you have to make cutbacks – look at this as a temporary situation. It is cathartic to strip back to bare essentials for a while. It will serve you well and help you appreciate money when you have more of it.

Step 2. Work on systematically paying off your debts. Everything other than a place to live, food, clothing, household bills and a means of transport should be viewed as a luxury. Stick to buying only essentials until your circumstances change. Work out a plan with your debtors to pay them off by a certain date. Do not borrow any more money or use credit cards.

Step 3. Let go of any worry or stress about financial matters. Avoid talking about your finances in a negative way as this will become a self-fulfilling mantra. Instead, accept your circumstances but think of these lean times as a short interlude in your abundant life journey.

Step 4. Start focusing on creating more wealth. Decide what you want and believe it will happen. Write down on a piece of paper the financial goals that you want to achieve and include a time frame.

Step 5. Create a clear belief that life is going to change for the better and that you are going to realize your goals. Read your list every day and recite the following affirmations on a daily basis and with feeling. Get into the habit of silently affirming the following phrases when you awaken, when you shower, when you are driving or any time throughout the day:

I deserve abundance and prosperity.
I am always in the right place at the right time.
Abundance flows freely and naturally to me.
All of my needs are constantly met.

Step 6. Be pro-active. Put yourself in the marketplace where you can attract more money into your life. If you are already in a full-time job, start a sideline that has potential. Only invest or borrow if you have tested the market and know there is a genuine future for your venture. When you are clear and decisive, others will respond to you positively. If working for yourself is not an option, apply for new jobs that will suit your lifestyle and fulfil your ambitions. If you are under-qualified then make a plan to achieve the qualifications you need.

Step 7. Believe that you deserve to be abundant and successful. When you believe this on a deep, unconscious level you are sending out a powerful statement of intent. Doors will begin to open for you and you will attract into your life just what you need to become more abundant.

Coping with career stress

'If you ask what is the single most important key to longevity I would have to say it is avoiding worry, stress and tension. And if you didn't ask me, I'd still have to say it.'

George F. Burns

If you suffer from stress at work, the important thing to do is make changes. Don't think you have to stay stuck in a rut, as there are always other options. If changing jobs is not an option, look at what you can do to improve things within your existing situation. If your workload is excessive then it is important to be organized and prioritize what is most important. Delegate the less important stuff, if you can. If you work long hours, balance this out with rest and relaxation. Ensure you take breaks and have a twenty-minute self-hypnosis session in the middle of each day, which will help you recharge and become more effective. If there is nowhere to relax, leave the office and go for a walk to get some fresh air and a different perspective. Exercise will always reduce stress.

If you are having problems with a colleague or boss and need to confront them, request a meeting to air your opinion. Before the meeting, create a trance state so that you can visualize a positive outcome. Imagine yourself in the room with your colleague and see the meeting going exactly as you want it to go, getting your point of view across clearly, negotiating effectively, and communicating your needs exceptionally well. See yourself at the end of the meeting feeling satisfied with the outcome. If you do this a few times first you will be amazed at how well you are able to negotiate when the time comes.

Make your workspace as comfortable and relaxing an environment as possible. Play soothing music on earphones, or at your desk. Use plants and candles, essential oils, soft colours, a comfortable chair, whatever it takes to create a space where you can face each new challenge with courage and strength. When you add each little step together they become a powerful holistic force in combating a stressful work environment.

We can't always choose whom we work with and it can be frustrating to spend forty hours or more a week with someone who is an energy drain. If you can't change the circumstances then you will need to change the way that you deal with them. That means not allowing them to affect you in a negative way. The following technique will help you do that.

Protecting yourself from negative or stressful people

Close your eyes and take a few slow, deep breaths. Allow yourself to become calm and take a moment to clear your mind. Now imagine you are surrounded by a white protective light. Visualize this protective energy field all around your body, as though you have stepped inside a white bubble.

Inside this bubble, you will feel completely safe and secure from any negative energy. If anyone criticizes you or is negative towards you, it will bounce off your protective shield and have no effect. Only positive thoughts and energy can pass through your protective light. The next time an adversarial colleague approaches, imagine you are inside your protective energy field, and they will no longer affect you in a negative way. You will feel completely different towards them and much more in control of your feelings.

Live in the
here and now

'Where does discontent start? You are warm enough, but you shiver. You are fed, yet hunger gnaws you. You have been loved, but your yearning wanders in new fields.'

John Steinbeck

Never yearn for things you don't have and avoid living in the future. Keep your focus on the here and now: when you visualize your abundant lifestyle see it as though it is in the present. Work on being more self-contained and do not rely on others for your well-being and happiness. You will become much stronger in this way and build your inner strength. This in turn begins to attract good things towards you. Work on your self and nurture the good in you. Be disciplined and focused while keeping your mind open and free.

Work on keeping your emotions in check with the ebb and flow of life. Don't get too carried away when you reach highs, or too down if you hit setbacks. If you have a few failures, avoid getting over-emotional. Just accept you have learnt a lesson and you won't make that error again. Overcoming problems and achieving your goals will happen if you work hard and put the effort in. You really can achieve anything when you focus your mind, and the limits as to what you achieve will be set by your own ambition.

Golden rule 5
financial security

- Debt is debilitating and will hold you back. Many people get seduced into buying the latest whatever on finance when they can't really afford it. Avoid such traps.

- Never focus on what you don't have. Set clear financial goals, print them out and put them in places where you will read and affirm them every day.

- Make a habit of believing success is your divine right. If you believe you will be financially secure and you take action to make it happen then you will create your own financial and career success.

Step 6

Relationships

'My religion is simple. My religion is kindness.'

Dalai Llama

Traditions and expectations

Fifty years ago families stayed in regular close contact. People generally married for life and, even when their children grew up and started their own families, they usually lived nearby so there was a reassuring sense of stability. It is when this stability and closeness breaks down that problems often begin, especially in times of crisis. Nowadays people are far more independent and have many more choices and options. Couples don't feel they have to stay stuck in unhappy marriages and may have children with more than one partner. The divorce rate is at an all-time high and it is common for children to be raised by a single parent or with an extra step-parent. Many old family traditions have been lost and forgotten, sabotaged by time or distance and replaced by the need for constant stimulation. For example, families don't always spend meal times together, which was once a vital time for cohesion and communication.

Relationships with loved ones and friends can become problematic if people don't live up to each other's expectations. If you think about those in your life who you have relationship problems with, the chances are those problems will have arisen because you believe they acted incorrectly in some way or vice versa. If you can adopt a more liberal attitude and allow people to be a pain in the arse now and again, it can help. If possible, sit down with the person you have the problem with and talk to them. Make sure the territory is neutral and there is no one else around. If this doesn't work, you can always go to a relationship counsellor who can help you get to the bottom of your unresolved issues with no pre-judgement.

The following mini-programme will give you some pointers to help you communicate effectively and, hopefully, heal the relationship. They are generalized and will not fit every situation, so adapt them for your own needs.

5 mini-steps to heal relationship conflicts

Step 1. Ask the person with whom you are in conflict if they would meet you to discuss the problem. It is preferable to work with one person at a time.

Step 2. Meet at a neutral public venue, like a pub or coffee bar that neither of you frequent and, preferably, equidistant from each of you. If you live in the same house, go for a walk together in an uplifting place like a woodland or park.

Step 3. Before the meeting, project a feeling of love towards the person. Even though this love may not be reciprocated, do not worry. Just send them a genuine feeling of unconditional love and try to hold on to that feeling throughout your discussions, even if you still disagree. It will help you to express yourself more positively and you will feel better for it afterwards.

Step 4. Greet them with a genuine compliment, such as 'You are looking well.' Start on a positive note and try to remain respectful throughout the meeting, even if it gets heated. When you talk, look them in the eye and stay strong and positive.

Step 5. If you have issues to get across, say them along these lines – 'I am really sorry we have got to this point and that we don't agree, but I am here because I genuinely want to get rid of the bad feeling between us. You may not like everything I have to say, but I am going to be honest and say how I feel, as I really want us to resolve our dispute and build a more positive relationship. Please hear me out before you make a judgement'. Then state your case with honesty and clarity and speak from your heart. When they speak, encourage them to speak from their heart too. Listen carefully to what they say and try to understand their point of view. This will help you build bridges and hopefully resolve the conflict.

Opening your heart and mind

'Children begin by loving their parents; as they grow older they judge them; sometimes they forgive them.'

Oscar Wilde

There is a great line in a classic song by The Doors that says, 'People are strange, when you're a stranger'. How often have you met someone and been put off by the way they spoke or looked, but warmed to them once you got to know them better? When you get into the habit of projecting out positive feelings to everyone you meet without prejudice, this will open your heart and you will change the way you feel towards others. You will become naturally more compassionate and loving and, importantly, you will become a magnet for attracting more love back into your life. This is a great technique for helping you to feel good inside and generally improve your relationships with people.

You still need to be aware, however, that no matter how loving you are there are some people who will not reflect that love back at you. Whenever you come across them, use the white light protection technique to avoid your energy being drained. Establish firm boundaries if you need to; don't be afraid to push them away if they are an energy drain. When you learn to love people it should come from a place of strength, not where you subjugate yourself. Be loving, compassionate and big-hearted, but at the same time be strong and never let others push you around. That is real strength.

Relationships between parents and children can be an area that causes not only a great deal of anxiety and stress, but that visibly ages the older generation. How many times have you heard a parent tell their child that they are giving them grey hairs? As family life has become fragmented, communication breakdowns are at the heart of many of these problems. Every town and city seems to have disaffected teenagers hanging around on street corners looking for trouble. I know because I was once one of them! This doesn't happen nearly so much in countries like Spain and Italy where the family unit still holds great importance and the matriarchal figures are strong. Fathers are often present, respected and communicative with their children. I am generalizing a bit here, but the bottom line is that, when parents are involved with their children and give them time, those children grow up well-balanced and better able to cope with life's challenges.

If you can communicate with your children at each step of their development, you will be able to influence their behaviour. It doesn't mean you will always like what they are doing, but if the channels are open then you'll at least have a hope of getting through to them. Talking to and understanding your kids are very important. You should never give up on them. If possible, make a habit of having at least one meal a day with your family or whomever you live with. Use that time to communicate and to resolve problems if you need to. Remember, positive communication is the key.

I never met a bad kid who didn't have incompetent parents. Bad parents are not always bad people; they often simply lack the understanding of their children's changing needs. In my hypnotherapy practice, I have had people bring their kids to me because they need help with problem behaviour, but the parents are almost always a big part of the problem. Whenever parents offer love, security and understanding, children prosper and flourish. I know it is not always easy to achieve this, especially in divorce or separation, but you should always put your kids first – before your ego, your needs and your wants. Even if your partner doesn't do the same, you should lead by example.

Sigmund Freud, one of the fathers of modern psychology, had some strange theories but also some extremely valid ones. One of his better notions was that children go through a number of specific stages of development in their journey from infancy to adulthood. If any of those stages are dysfunctional or problematic then a part of the child becomes psychologically stuck at that stage of their development. The next time you see an adult acting like a child, you can bet it is the child part of them acting up. We are very subtle beings and our childhood conditioning creates behaviour blueprints that remain with us for the rest of our adult lives.

It is possible to overcome destructive patterns in adult life through various therapies. In my hypnotherapy work I always found that regressing people to the root cause of the problem is a powerful way to release and overcome destructive patterns of behaviour, fears and anxieties. Imagine, though, how great it would be if we could avoid

Relationships case study

When I split from my first wife, we were in our mid-twenties and my son was a baby. However, we both agreed to set our differences aside and put our child first. My wife moved back to her mother's house and we lived fifty miles apart, but I made the one-hundred-mile round trip at least once a week for well over ten years, without fail. Even though I was broke then and my cars weren't always up to the trip, I never missed a week. I was always welcomed by my ex-wife and her family and enjoyed great communication with my son through every step of his childhood.

I also made the most of the time I had with him, as it was precious. Although my son grew up in a single-parent household, he is now a well-balanced, positive young man with a million-and-one plans for his future. I am still great friends with my ex-wife and I continue to support her, as she has been a wonderful mother to my son. She even comes on holidays with me, my son and my wife. It is a bit weird going away with two wives, but they are good friends and people often say how nice this is. Although we divorced, we put our egos aside and worked hard to give our son an example of how to have a good relationship in spite of our differences.

passing problems on to our children in the first place. If the next generation of parents were truly enlightened, if every father was strong and disciplined but also compassionate and sensitive and every mother was nurturing, caring, loving and always put her children's needs first, they would give their children huge self-belief and confidence. They would teach them to be respectful, positive, independent and live life to the full. If we could collectively achieve this in a single generation we would wipe out delinquency, crime, conflict, maybe even war. A little idealistic, I know, but why not strive to do your bit and take your parenting skills up another level? Being a parent is one of the most underrated jobs in the world, yet the rewards are huge. In the fullness of your lifetime, your parenting efforts will far outweigh the rewards of a good career or making money.

If you are in a situation where your relationship with your partner is the problem, try to use the advice given earlier to improve communication and open up channels of love and understanding. Even if this feels difficult, give it a go. Sometimes the path of least resistance is the best one. It takes two people to have a fight and turning the other cheek is often the best response. I am not suggesting you become submissive, but if there is conflict and dispute, try to rise above it. Act with honesty and integrity even if the other person does not. There is a real strength in acting that way when

7 mini-steps to improve your parenting skills

Step 1. Children need guidance and boundaries. They may not know or realize it, but they will feel more secure when they have rules to adhere to. You, as their parent, are their teacher. By giving them clear boundaries as to what is right or wrong, you are teaching them acceptable behaviour and respect. They will feel much more secure when you show strength and guidance.

Step 2. Whenever you set a boundary always explain the reason behind it. Speak with respect and compassion, but at the same time be firm. If you want to get your child into a positive behaviour pattern tell them positive stories about yourself when you were their age. Kids love stories, and will relate to yours. It will also help them to understand you, where you came from and why you are asking them to behave in a certain way.

Step 3. One of the best things you can give your children is a strong feeling of self-belief. From day one, always encourage your children and let them believe they can achieve anything. Kids have unlimited imaginations. With encouragement they will prosper and flourish throughout their lives. Tell them often that they are good, clever, smart, funny, bright and talented and that is what they will become. Pick your moments and impart your praise in the right context. Never underestimate the power of your words.

Step 4. Never use destructive language when speaking to your children. Kids are like sponges and absorb everything. If you make a habit of telling them they are useless, stupid or hopeless, that will become self-fulfilling. So cut any such language from your vocabulary when you speak to them and never shout at them. If they play up, always count to ten before telling them in a firm and controlled way how you want them to behave. If you need to assert your authority, send them to their rooms or whatever means of enforcement you prefer.

Step 5. Have fun with your kids. Children of all ages thrive on adventure. If you get into the habit of playing with them, you will build a strong bond with them that will last for life. Make this a habit through every stage of their development. There is nothing more liberating than being silly with your kids. It will connect you to a carefree fun part of yourself.

Step 6. Children go through many growth stages, physically and emotionally. At some stage, they may begin to distance themselves from you or become obnoxious, rebellious and argumentative. When this occurs, don't judge them. Give them some space and try to understand the cause of these changes in their behaviour, which is a natural breaking away to form their own identity. It is healthy and should be encouraged. They will always come back to you if the bonds are strong. So handle them carefully and cut them some slack.

Step 7. Let your kids know you love them. You may think they already know, but they will believe and accept it more readily when you actually say it to them. Children thrive on love and security and you can't give them enough of it. Get into the habit of saying 'I love you' so that it becomes the norm and is not an embarrassment. This will also help them to know that you are proud of them. Nurturing and empowering your kids are the most important things you will do in your life, without question

faced with hostility. In the end, you will feel better for not lowering yourself to the level of others. In subsequent relationships you will attract partners towards you who are like you, so cultivating positive ethics and a big-hearted attitude in the face of conflict is good for your soul.

The following is a wonderful tool to help you improve relationships. It will also help you develop more compassion for others and, ultimately, for yourself.

Big-heartedness

Take a moment to get in a comfortable position, then close your eyes and focus on your breathing. Begin to breathe very slowly and deeply: in through your nose and out through your mouth. Make each breath long and deep, feel your rib cage expand as you breathe in. Continue this for a short while until all the tension disappears from your body, and you feel nice and relaxed.

Now imagine you are surrounded by a pure white light. See and feel this protective white light all around you, filling your aura. In this special place, allow yourself to feel very secure and calm. Become aware of your heart beating in your chest with a strong and steady rhythm, and imagine your heart is filled with pure white light. See the purity of the light and know that this resonates with unconditional love. It may be the kind of love a mother feels for her baby or a father for his child. Take a moment to feel this special white light of love growing brighter and brighter.

Now visualize the light expanding out from your heart so that it begins to fill your whole body. As you do so, begin to connect with feelings of compassion and love for all things. Continue to imagine the light expanding, filling your entire body and spreading out into your aura. Then imagine it expanding further still, as though this spark of light has grown so strong that it now projects out and away from you in every direction. Connect with this deep feeling of love and compassion growing stronger and stronger as the white light grows ever brighter, as it reaches further and further.

Imagine your white light of unconditional love reaching out and engulfing others: maybe people you know or those you want to reach. Feel a strong feeling of love for these people and deep compassion for their struggles and troubles. See their faults and weaknesses as manifestations of difficulties in their life. As you continue to imagine the white light illuminating everything before you and expanding ever further, connect now with a feeling of love and compassion, knowledge and personal power. At this point, you can also repeat some affirmations to compound this feeling of love and compassion. State your affirmations as a reality now in the present tense. Here are some examples, but please adapt and add your own to suit your needs:

> **I love to develop positive relationships with people.**
> **I am compassionate and understanding.**
> **I give and receive love easily.**
>
> When you state your affirmations, draw the words inside you and really believe them. As always, you will need to practise the technique a few times and repeat the affirmations regularly to get the best results. Stay in this moment for a short time so you can continue to reach out with your unconditional love. Then, when you are ready, count from one to three: 1 ... 2 ... 3 .... Open your eyes and come back to full waking consciousness.

There is a saying, 'What goes around comes around', and with relationships that is never more true. Whatever you give out to those around you comes back at you. Love breeds love, impatience engenders impatience, and so on. When you are thinking about your relationship with another person, especially if it is a difficult one, imagine yourself in their shoes for a moment. See things from their perspective and think how they must be feeling. Only then will you see that they, too, have a point of view that they are fully entitled to, or that you may not always be right, or qualified to judge or advise them.

Keep an open heart and allow only positive energy

into it. Send that positive, forgiving, healing energy back out and immediately you will notice a difference in your relationships. By removing the stress and angst of tricky situations with loved ones, or those you have to live and work with, you are freeing your mind to concentrate on the things that really matter, and on your own health and happiness.

Golden rule 6 relationships

- To improve your relationships with others the change has to start from within you. It is not always easy but if you are willing to make a shift within yourself you can go a long way to creating good relationships with people.

- The universal law of attraction states that whatever you project out will come back to you. When you feel love and compassion for others, you will naturally attract love and compassion back to you.

- Work on one relationship at a time. Think of a person that you want to improve your relationship with. Close your eyes, take a few breaths and let go of any grievance or hurt and simply project feelings of love and compassion towards them. Have an understanding of their struggles and journey in life. Imagine a strong feeling of love coming from your heart and reaching their heart, and silently focus on the word 'love'. When you do this, avoid judgement or discrimination, just focus on feeling love, compassion and understanding. Practise this often with those you come into contact with and all your relation-ships will improve.

Step 7

Spritual well-being

'Your vision will become clear only when you look
    into your heart.
Who looks outside, dreams. Who looks inside,
    awakens.'

Carl Jung

Embracing life and the ageing process

Spiritual well-being is as important as a positive mental
attitude, if not more so. Unless you are happy within
your spiritual self and feel completely in harmony
with your environment and the mind and body you are
blessed with then happiness will elude you, and with it,
long life and good health.

Many people are fearful of getting older, especially
in a generation where youth and physical perfection are

increasingly portrayed as so important. The ageing process should be embraced as a natural part of life, not as something that causes stress. Some people become more fearful and even reclusive with age. It doesn't help that the elderly are often not respected in the way that they should be. Many cultures hold their elders in high esteem, but in the West we seem to have lost this tradition.

People also fret about their health as they age, without realizing that they have the power to make positive changes to become healthier, no matter what their age. The older generation, in particular, has been indoctrinated into believing that modern medicine has the answers and is suspicious of alternative therapies or courses of action. Yet modern medicine often only treats symptoms, without curing the disease. A healthy diet and a positive, healthy mind coupled with a toned and fit body will prevent the onset of almost all illness and disease. It really is that simple, but then life is often far simpler than people realize when you get it right. So keep working on achieving that simplicity through making as many small positive changes as you can.

Working on your mental, spiritual and physical fitness will undoubtedly slow the ageing process. Part of that, especially if you have health concerns, is to stop worrying and be proactive. When I was twenty years old, I could spend the weekend boozing, smoking and

Ageing case study

A man in his eighties bought one of my books and some of my recordings and decided he simply had to come and see me in person. As he lived many miles away, this involved him taking four train journeys and a cab ride. When he arrived, he told me he was studying for a degree at his local university, but was having difficulty remembering his coursework, something that annoyed him intensely. I was amazed at his positive attitude and his determination to keep improving his mind at what surely had to be the tail-end of his long life. His frustration at what he saw as his personal weakness was the only bitter element of his conversation.

Through hypnosis, I was able to open up his mind to the better retention of information, thereby improving his memory and mental stamina. With his approval, I was also able to encourage him to accept his physical limitations as part of the natural ageing process and not get so frustrated with himself. I reinforced all the good that he was doing by keeping physically and mentally active and by the end of our sessions, he was much happier and felt less judgmental of himself. He wrote to me some months later to inform me that he had not only passed his degree, he had passed with distinction!

partying all night long and still wake up on Monday morning looking good. If I carried on like that now, I'd look like a bloated old vagrant in no time. It is a fact of life that you have to work a little harder to remain vibrant and healthy as you get older. You can enjoy doing just that through your visualizations and all the techniques you have learned in this book so far. When you create a healthy holistic lifestyle, it soon becomes addictive. A positive addiction is fine, as long as it doesn't go to extremes.

There is nothing wrong with wanting to slow the ageing process, but it is important to keep it in balance. Don't obsess about ageing or get down about the way your face and body change as you grow older. It happens to everyone – rich, poor or famous. Having a positive attitude will help you to adapt to these changes and accept that growing old it is not a stressful concept. If you still have a problem accepting the way you look, the following technique will help. It may not be easy at first, as you are trying to change your perception and create a more positive feeling of self-acceptance. The way to approach this is to view it as though you are re-programming your mind to feel more positive about yourself.

They say there are three perceptions of one's self: our own, other peoples', and the real one. If you feel better about yourself and the way you look, you will come across as a more positive person and, as a by-product, you will appear more attractive to others. So, when using this technique, use the 'fake it until you make it' principle, even if it feels awkward at first. If you can scale the heights and love yourself unconditionally, other people will become more loving towards you. Whatever the inner you projects outwards will affect the way people respond to you.

Accepting yourself and the way you look

Go to a quiet room and look at your face in the mirror. Examine it closely and accept yourself as you are, with any lines or imperfections. Take a few deep breaths and relax and clear your mind of any conscious thought. Aim to create a feeling of complete relaxation through your breathing and mental focus. Then project a strong feeling of love and acceptance as you stare at your face and into your eyes.

Repeat to yourself, 'I love and accept myself'. Use your feelings.

Project a feeling of love, compassion and acceptance for who you are and the way you look. Make the feelings very positive and continue this habit on a daily basis.

New way of thinking

'Life is a series of experiences, each of which makes
us bigger, even though it is hard to realize this.'

Henry Ford

The key to your success is in re-programming your old
thought patterns. If you can exercise regularly, eat
healthily and feel happy and contented with your life,
you will knock years off you. It is as simple as that.
Now imagine this is easy to do, as though it is second
nature to you. Imagine you have no desire for your old,
unhealthy, discontented lifestyle. You are slim and fit
and the best you can possibly be. You no longer crave
sweets, fries, fizzy drinks or fattening foods. You enjoy
drinking plenty of water, taking exercise and love how it
is toning and shaping your body. You sleep soundly every
night, feel happy and positive, are free from stress over
financial or career worries and enjoy healthy relationships with all you know and love. You can easily live
a perfectly happy life without ever worrying about it
again. This is an easy mindset to create and I will show
you how.

Do you remember the first time you learned a new
skill, for example the first time you got into a car and
learned to drive? For almost everyone, learning to

change gear and pull away smoothly was a difficult experience at first. In time it became easier. Then after plenty of practice, you found you could move easily through the gears without any conscious thought. Now driving is an automatic, unconscious process. You can use that same inherent learning ability to teach yourself to love everything about your new healthy life. You can learn to enjoy feeling fit and find all that was harmful to you before abhorrent. Whatever your personal aims, you can re-programme your mind in specific ways to help you to achieve your goals. Learning these new habits is a matter of repetition and compounding. The more you visualize and absorb the affirmations you need, the quicker you create the new inner belief. It is also enjoyable as you will be creating relaxing mental states, which will benefit your general health and well-being.

Finding courage

'Shoot for the moon. Even if you miss, you'll land among the stars.'

Anon

It is healthy to step out of our comfort zones now and again. Doing so helps focus the mind on the lives we lead and look at them from a whole new perspective. Like going away on holiday, when we 'come back' from these experiences, we often appreciate what we have with new vision and clarity, and are able to see what, if anything, needs to change for us to feel more contented.

On your journey to a younger, healthier you, there will be times when you are faced with big dilemmas and will need to make bold decisions. Finding the courage to face these decisions and make the right choice can be daunting. You may be faced with a decision as insignificant as whether or not to head to the gym one night or to go down the pub with your mates instead. Or it may be something much deeper and more problematical, such as whether to cut ties with a friend, partner or relative who is an energy drain and is holding you back from your goals. Your visualizations and affirmations will help with all of these decisions, but sometimes you may feel you need to draw on something a bit stronger, to give you the faith you need.

Experiences like fire walking, bungee jumping, rock climbing or freefall can be great for boosting confidence and self-esteem. If you walk across burning hot coals or throw yourself off a cliff with just a piece of rubber attached to your ankle, it leaves you with a feeling that you can take on anything in life. Of course, daredevil adventures may not be for you and you may prefer to try something less dangerous. Whatever it is that takes you out of your usual habits and routines to a place where you feel that – for you – this is a risk, I guarantee it will prove to be a life-enhancing and often life-changing experience for your spiritual and physical self.

I once took part in a North American Indian ceremony that involved a small group of people sitting for hours in a tent or tepee, known as a 'sweat lodge'. Hot stones were placed on a fire in the centre of the mud floor of the tent so that the heat became intense. The aim was to cleanse the body of toxins, the mind of negatives and to heighten the spirit. My sweat lodge experience was an all-male affair in the middle of remote English countryside on the December day of the Winter Solstice. Ten of us stood around as naked as the day we were born, freezing winds whistling around our private parts, while a short ceremony took place. We then spent the next four hours in the sauna-like conditions of the tent meditating and getting to know each other. The idea was to break down barriers and to connect with our inner spirits. We were from all walks of life – middle-aged businessmen, tree-huggers, some New Age chaps with dreadlocks and a few ordinary working men.

As part of the process, we each had to ask for one thing and meditate on this as a personal goal. One of the men asked for greater knowledge, one asked for compassion, and another asked for happiness. When it came to my turn, I asked to be financially rich. My response was greeted with shock and even opposition from some of my fellow tepee occupiers. Several thought it was not 'spiritual' to make such a request and we were soon embroiled in a lively debate. I pointed out that when I became rich I planned to use it for good, to help others and experience life more fully. I am sure a couple of them thought me shallow and crass in my request and they were, of course, entitled to their opinion.

I honestly believed then, as I still believe now, that having money has helped me develop my spirituality and made me a better person. There is no bigger kick for me than to help out a friend or family member who needs a financial leg-up or to donate spontaneously to a worthy cause that touches me. As a result of my hypnosis audios selling in large numbers, I have started a company and employed others to help them achieve happiness and stability in their own lives. Furthermore, I have travelled around the world and become more knowledgeable and enlightened as a result. I believe I have acted, throughout, with integrity and honesty. What is "unspiritual" about any of that? There is no exclusive spirituality in poverty.

Releasing fear

'The only thing we have to fear is fear itself –
nameless, unreasoning, unjustified terror which
paralyzes needed efforts to convert retreat into
advance.'

Franklin D. Roosevelt

I once watched an astronaut speaking on a documentary
about his view of the Earth from the Apollo rocket taking
him to the Moon. He said that he only realized how
insignificant he was when he looked back at our tiny
blue planet, suspended like a ball in the blackness of the
universe, defenceless, alone and – in the overall scheme
of things – apparently unimportant to the rest of space.
Raising his thumb and closing one eye, he could blot
Earth out of his vision altogether. 'After that, I vowed to
never take myself too seriously again,' he said, with a wry
smile.

We sometimes forget how insignificant we are. Tiny
ants, crawling on the surface of a little blue ball in the
middle of some distant galaxy; each of us believing we
are the centre of the universe and that everything that
happens to us happens for a reason and is felt as keenly
by those around us. Yes, of course, each of us matters and
has the divine right to be on this Earth, to live, love and

enjoy life to the best of our abilities. That is what this book is all about – making the most of our time here, fulfilling our potential and creating a healthy mind and body to inhabit for as long as we possibly can. But when you don't connect with yourself spiritually, when you start to focus on what is happening around you rather than what is happening within you, you can often lose your way.

It isn't hard these days to have our attention drawn to the bad things about this world. Wars, famine, oppression, recession, greed, cruelty – all assail our senses daily in news reports and bulletins that can, if we let them, grind us down and force us to lose sight of all the good in the world. Fear sets in – of impending doom or catastrophe, worries about situations completely beyond our control. The trick is not to buy into that fear. I have treated so many people for a pathological fear of flying – usually sparked by watching graphic news stories or documentaries about plane crashes – when, statistically, flying is one of the safest forms of travel. Irrational fear stifles them to the point that they cannot function and sometimes can't even go near an airport. Yet, by using a simple self-hypnosis technique they can easily overcome the fear, move forward and live life to the full again, taking foreign holidays with friends and families once more.

Fear case study

A woman who was about to be married came to me with an irrational anxiety of flying. She had never had this fear until she met her fiancé, who was so afraid of flying that he would suffer panic attacks if he even saw an aeroplane on television. She desperately wanted to go to Thailand for their honeymoon, but did not think she could cope with the journey as on their previous flight together they had both endured feelings of extreme anxiety. Her hope was that if I could help her, her fiancé would also come to see me and they could have the honeymoon of their dreams. In her late twenties, she seemed completely rational about everything else, so I was sure I would be able to help her with her problem.

In our first session together, I hypnotized her easily and took her to a calm and tranquil state where I walked her through the journey she was about to make, from the moment she left home until the time she disembarked from the aeroplane in Thailand. By desensitizing her to the perceived stresses of the journey, I was able to run through the entire experience with the suggestion that she feel positive and calm throughout, and thoroughly enjoy the experience. The session went very well and, after two further sessions, she assured me she was no longer afraid of flying.

A few days later her fiancé came to see me, as she had hoped. Sitting in front of me with his arms folded defensively across his chest, he made it quite clear that he didn't believe in hypnotherapy and didn't think I could help him. Believing I would have my work cut out, I was surprised when he fell into a trance state very quickly and was able to recount how his fear of flying stemmed from his father's nervous disposition and a plane journey the two of them had taken when he was a boy. Two sessions later the fiancé, too, was free of his anxiety. They sent me a postcard from their Thai honeymoon to thank me and to tell me how much they had enjoyed their journey.

Six months later, I bumped into the woman on a street corner and asked her how things were. 'You won't believe it!' she told me, laughing. 'He's gone from one extreme to the other. He's taken up bungee jumping, hang-gliding and is about to do his first parachute jump! I don't know what you did to him but he's a changed man.' I couldn't imagine what I had said or done to trigger such a keen interest in dangerous sports, but as the two of them seemed thrilled, I was happy too.

What this story illustrates so well, and is important never to forget, is that you have unlimited power and potential inside you. This man who could barely see a plane on television is now living life to the full and enjoying being released from a fear that stemmed from his childhood. Once you have released any conditioning that has disempowered you, the world is your oyster!

The following technique will help.

Blue sky thinking

Get yourself into a comfortable position, close your eyes and start your deep breathing until you feel completely relaxed. Allow your mind to go completely blank. Imagine you are looking up at the sky on a pleasant summer's day. You notice a few small clouds that drift across the sky and then fade away. These are your unwanted thoughts and the visual manifestations of the bad conditioning that has previously disempowered you. See these manifestations for what they are – clouds of vapour that have no real substance. Tell yourself not to fear them, as they will soon drift away. Every time you see a cloud or get an unwanted thought, imagine it disappearing and your mind becoming clear. Eventually all of the clouds have drifted away and the sky is completely clear. Imagine your conscious thought as this clear blue backdrop to the perfect sky.

Connecting with your higher self

'The life of inner peace, being harmonious and without stress, is the easiest type of existence.'

Norman Vincent Peale

Sometimes it can help to give problems up to your higher powers or whatever force you believe is guiding you through life. So, when you have a problem or are beset by fears, always create time to switch off and go inside yourself and ask for guidance. Affirm that the solution will come to you when you need it. You may be just asking your inner self for guidance, or those with traditional religious or more alternative beliefs may feel drawn to ask those they think are guiding them through this earthly life.

Connecting with yourself and your spiritual inner being in this way, or any way you feel appropriate, will reinforce all the lessons you have learned on your journey and help you to continue on your chosen path. Never underestimate the power of these meditations and visualization techniques. Repeated affirmations compound the beliefs you have chosen to endorse and, even if you are not fully aware of their influence on you, will continue to work in your unconscious mind and guide you on your quest.

Connecting with your higher self

Take a moment to get in a comfortable position, close your eyes and focus on your breathing. Once again, begin to breathe deeply and slowly, in through your nose and out through your mouth, creating a circular breathing motion. At the top of your breath hold it for three seconds: 1 ... 2 ... 3 ... then silently and mentally count to five on every out-breath: 1 ... 2 ... 3 ... 4 ... 5 ... As you breathe out, let go of any tension left in your body.

As you lie there relaxing more and more, imagine you are gazing up into the night sky. You notice many bright and beautiful stars. As you marvel at this wonderful picture you notice one particular star shining brightly, more than all the others: a shimmering glowing star, shining so brightly in the night sky, radiating energy and light. Your whole attention is drawn to this star. You feel there is something special about it, as though it is there to help you in some way. You sense that this star holds the key to everything you need to know to help you go forward successfully in life. This star will guide you and bring you knowledge.

Become completely focused on the tiny, white ball of light and notice it coming nearer but still remaining the size

of a tiny ball. See it come closer and closer until it is
hovering just above the crown of your head. Imagine it
floating in mid-air above your head. You may at this point
feel a slight tingling sensation or a warm, comforting glow.

Feel a part of you is in this special light – the spirit part
of you that knows your life journey and vocation, the infinite
wisdom part of you that is your higher self. Now draw this
ball of light inside you so that you are filled with understanding and knowledge. Affirm to yourself:

I have great wisdom and understanding.
I am aware and enlightened.
I understand my journey in life.

When you are ready, slowly count from one to ten,
and open your eyes and come back to full waking
consciousness.

Golden rule 7
spiritual well-being

- We all have busy lives that consume us and make us feel important at times. Remember that you are one of six billion inhabiting a tiny planet in a small galaxy in billions of galaxies. Our sun is just one of billions of stars in universe so infinite we can't even begin to comprehend it.

- If you worry about the bad things that happen in this world – war, oppression, famine, corruption, evil – remember that the planet we live on is incredibly beautiful and has many wonders. The dark of the world may co-exist with the light but it is the light that throws the darkness into the shade.

- We live in a time of tremendous change. We can experience the whole gamut of our existence – the good, the bad and everything in between. The world is as it is and we are here to experience its extremes. We can, through our free will, make the world a better place. This in turn helps our own evolution and is our reason for being here – to learn and evolve.

- Each of us has embarked on a hazardous and heroic journey, but one with the potential for tremendous growth. With our free will we can become more complete beings with the knowledge we acquire.

- Have a higher meaning in your life. Viewing daily dramas from a bigger perspective will bring you inner peace. It will empower you and help you to move forward with a greater understanding. Make time to view the bigger picture more often.

- Do not obsess about growing old. It is all part of the natural cycle and should be embraced. Remain open to change, seek joy in simplicity and spiritual satisfaction, and continue on your quest to live long and happy, healthy in mind, body and spirit.

Look younger and live longer

I hope this book has inspired you to embark on a new path towards better health and happiness. There is no quick fix to looking younger and living longer, but you will be surprised how soon the changes start to show if you follow my seven steps.

My goal has been to help you create a holistic approach to achieving your goals by using many small building blocks and a few major therapy techniques. By now you should have embraced many of the changes and be well on the way to a new you. I sincerely hope this is the case. This whole journey must be something that you really enjoy, as you take back control of your life and adopt a new positive approach to fitness and diet and exercise and sleep, stress, your career and your mental and spiritual well-being.

If you learn to love being fit and healthy, sleeping soundly and freeing yourself from cares, everything else will fall into place. Friends and family will start noticing the difference in you almost immediately. This should reinforce your determination still further to carry on with your inner programming, until you have achieved the goals you have set yourself.

When you work on your affirmations, use the techniques and listen to the audio download regularly, this will become your new reality. You will develop a core belief about yourself and the way you want to be until you find yourself in complete control of all aspects of your life and that will feel intensely satisfying to you. So, keep immersing your inner mind with positive programming and you will achieve your goals. I wish you every success.

Further information

For a current list of my titles, contact:

Diviniti Publishing Ltd
Unit 1 Bourne Enterprise Centre
Wrotham Road
Borough Green
Kent
TN15 8DG
Telephone: 01732 882057
Email: sales@hypnosisaudio.com

My CDs and downloads can be purchased from
www.hypnosisaudio.com and my personal website
is www.glennharrold.com